And Beneath It
All Was Love

And Beneath It All Was Love

My Path Back Home Again Through Breast Cancer

A Memoir

Aime Alley Card

ISBN: 0692592466
ISBN 13: 9780692592465
Library of Congress Control Number: 2016901433
Aime A Card, Wenham, MA

For Scott, Catherine and Wesley
My love, my life

Table of Contents

Prologue

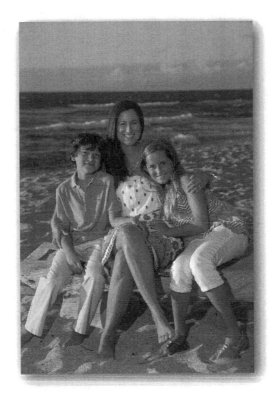

By the time a person reaches her forties, chances are she's had a friend who's been treated for cancer. Probably more than one. Mostly the friends just disappear then reemerge in a few months with different hair, maybe looking a little thinner and more tired.

I am that friend. I wanted to disappear. But now I want you to see what it was like. What it was really like. Not the *I'm fine* that I would normally give you, or the upbeat take on the latest reports from the doctor, but the real deal. This is what happened last year behind the walls that I put up to protect myself.

I am concerned that I was one of those people who appeared on the outside to sail through it. I want to be clear. No one who goes through chemotherapy sails through it. It's brutal. But most of us quietly go about the business of healing and "pull in" to deal with it. I hate laying my problems out for people. I hate admitting vulnerability. But I will do it now because I think it is important for people to know what happens behind the closed doors. We did our best. That's all anyone can do in a situation like this. And we made it. The four of us. Together.

CHAPTER 1

❧

The Beginning
February

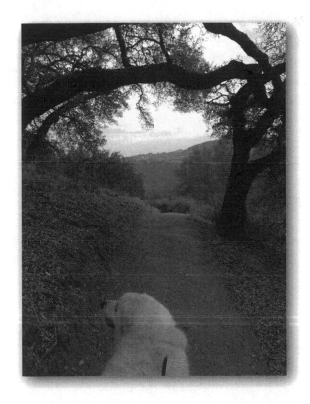

MAVERICK, A HUGE white furry mass of a dog, bounded happily out of the car in the parking lot at Pulgas Ridge. He tugged eagerly against his leash while I said hello to Lauren and we started up the path.

"Oh my gosh, he's so excited," she said and laughed at him as he kept a few feet ahead of us, his nose roaming over everything in his path and tail swinging back and forth in a happy curl.

"He's been desperate to get out of the new house. He doesn't really love the yard. It's so steep and has all these prickly leaves," I said as we started our way up the trail.

"Oh, I know, what are those leaves? I know they're from the oak trees, but they're almost like holly leaves. It's so weird." Lauren kept up a quick pace beside me, swiveling her lean frame around the stray branches that crept onto the path.

Lauren and I had bonded immediately the previous summer when I called her to introduce myself as the room parent for the second grade class at school. Within five minutes we discovered that we were not only both East Coast transplants to Silicon Valley for our husbands' work in Tech Finance but also both originally from the South, both alumnae of the same college, and both women who had shocked their families by marrying boys from the northeast. Some family members called them Yankees, a term that always surprised Scott when he heard it and felt compelled to remind people that he was a Red Sox fan.

"Elizabeth came home from school yesterday and told me they had beta tested an app in class." Lauren shook her head, and her long red ponytail caught the sun for a moment.

I laughed. "I know, Wesley mentioned it too. I was impressed and horrified at the same time."

"When are they writing?" she asked, her voice rising. "With pencils? On paper?" She sidestepped around a stray prickly branch that crept into the path, her sneaker slipping a bit on the dry earth. We took a sharp turn in the path and I hopped up a couple of logs that had been laid across the path for extra support.

"At least if they start learning to code they can get jobs when they graduate," I said and pushed my long dark hair back off of my face, my fingers catching for a moment in a tangle before I pulled them free. I tugged an elastic band off my wrist and gathered my hair into a messy bun in one fluid movement.

Lauren laughed and nodded in agreement.

The irony of worrying about the tech emersion while catching up over a hike was not lost on me. In Northern California we enjoyed a rich outdoor life year round, but even the sporting seemed intense. People didn't just ride their bikes; they donned full-on Tour de France gear as they climbed over mountains and through towns in teams of thirty or more. They didn't just go for a walk; they had to hike Windy Hill, a hill that climbed steadily at a steep pitch for an hour all the way up to the mountain ridge at Skyline. It was work hard, play hard, but the main undercurrent that ran through the entire valley was Tech. The place breathed it. It seemed to permeate the air. Fortunes were risked and made daily from it. It was the modern day gold rush, and everyone wanted a piece of the gold.

We arrived at the crest of the ridge and rested for a few minutes, taking in the vast view over the canyons.

"Where are we?" Lauren asked, "I'm so turned around."

I followed her gaze toward the far ridge and said, "That is the back side of Devonshire Canyon, where we live, and just through there you can see the bay." I pointed between the two ridgelines where the white patches from the salt banks in the bay caught my attention.

"It's cool over here. I do miss Woodside, being so close to school and most of our friends, and how quiet it is. But this is good too," I said.

I glanced down at Maverick resting by my feet. Sensing my attention, he rolled over on his back, exposing his great white belly and giving me a goofy grin in anticipation of a good scratch. I laughed at him and indulged him, giving the warm area under his foreleg a vigorous rub. He let out a deep groan of appreciation.

Our first two years in California had been spent in a large but dilapidated old house at the base of King's Mountain in Woodside. The previous spring the owner decided to cash out on his investment while the market was hot, so we had to scramble to find a new rental. We had been one of multiple applicants for the one place within half an hour of the kids' school in Menlo Park, and we were lucky we had gotten it.

"It really is beautiful here. We wouldn't be hiking like this in February in New Jersey," Lauren said, seeming to enjoy the quiet moment.

"Certainly not in Boston, either." I said. "So how's the benefit coming along?"

Lauren had been drafted to take on a big role in the school's primary fundraiser because of her social media and marketing background. The committee had been working for a couple of months and Lauren had expressed some frustration at what she described as a lack of direction from the committee. The president had happily described herself as "not a micro-manager, but a delegator," to which Lauren had responded, "that is fine except that I won't know what you need me to do unless you ask for it."

I felt sympathetic to Lauren and to the president. I'd been in both roles before, so I knew how these committees could go. It was a lot of busy mothers with high-level degrees and business experience channeling their talents into one big splashy event. The pressure was on each year to be better than the year before—to raise more money and to make this the year that people remembered. The result was an exponential increase of extravagance from year to year that a team of unpaid volunteers struggled to manage.

I had bowed out of leadership that year, taking on the simple task of catalog writing, so I could focus on a blog that I was building as a resource for new families settling into Silicon Valley, but I still enjoyed hearing about the latest plans and how things were going.

"Ugh." Lauren rolled her eyes and made a grunting sound. "It's a lot of hassle and chaos right now. You're so glad you're not in those meetings every week."

"I'm sure it will all come together in the end. It always does. Ready to head down?" I asked, getting up and brushing the dirt off my leggings.

"Let's go." Lauren said, hopping up and stretching her long thin legs side to side.

We started back down the edge of the ridge at a leisurely pace, following a path that was cut into the side of a steep incline. A red-tailed hawk circled and called overhead, and I watched it glide gracefully along with the wind. Maverick ambled along slowly, and Lauren and I fell back into conversation, alternating between being single file and side-by-side on the trail.

"Oh, did I tell you? I'm on a paleo diet now," Lauren said. "Basically you eat like a caveman. Whatever the early humans were able to gather or kill. Mostly nuts, greens, seeds, some fruit, meat, fish and seafood."

"Wow. That's pretty intense." I shook my head. "I'm just trying to limit processed food as much as I can. Although I don't think I'll ever get the kids to give up Goldfish." I debated for a moment, then decided to fess up. "I have to get control of my health. I have a biopsy tomorrow, and it's making me nervous."

"Oh no, what's going on?" she asked, slowing her pace a little and looking at me.

"A little cluster of spots showed up on my mammogram last week and they want to check it out. I'm sure it's nothing."

We wound our way back to the bottom of the ridge and said our goodbyes in the parking lot, and as Maverick took a bounding jump into the back of the car, Lauren waved and called out, "Good luck with everything, I'll be thinking about you!"

The biopsy was a fairly simple procedure, and while I waited for the results I remembered what the surgeon had told me when I asked her how often the results she saw were positive. She looked me straight in the eye and said, "Eighty percent of the biopsies I do are negative, so hold onto that, okay?"

Two days later, I sat in my doctor's office. The biopsy surgeon had said she would call within five to eight days with the full analysis, that she didn't bother with preliminaries because in her estimation it was best to have all the information at once. My general practitioner didn't abide by that philosophy, and I gratefully sat while he called the lab for the initial results, which were ultimately the most important, I thought. Positive or negative. As I watched, I heard a terse medical conversation take place. The only clear words I heard were "stage two."

He hung up the phone and looked at me.

"Well, the news isn't good. It is positive. You do have cancer. But it is early and treatments these days have greatly improved." He let that sink in for a moment while I blinked at him, then he continued, "The first step is to get lined up with a surgeon. I will find out who the best at Stanford is and give you a referral. The referral network can be slow over there, so I suggest you also call to make an appointment to expedite the process."

We talked for a few more minutes over the details and I stood, finished, ready to escape and go sit in my car alone. He ushered me out and wished me good luck. He was officially passing the baton.

I made it out to my car before I fell apart. I left a message for Scott and then, not ready to talk to anyone else, I started group texting my sisters.

Aime: It was positive. Can you call Dad and Rob?
Lea: Okay. What's the plan.
Aime: Lumpectomy. As soon as possible.
Lea: Caught it early right?
Emma: Okay. Will they wait until after that to decide anything else?
Lea: Let me know if you feel like talking. I'll call them now.
Aime: Sorry, I just need some time to process.
Emma: So it's just a small spot?
Aime: Yes, a small cluster.
Lea: They will take good care of you!!

Emma: Absolutely! They've made so many advances and this part wasn't so bad for mom.

Aime: Yes. Scott is out of town, of course.

Emma: Let us know if you need anything or need to talk. Do you have the kids?

Aime: Not yet. I'm about to go get them. I don't know what to say to anyone.

Emma: Just wait until you're ready.

Lea: I'm sorry he's not there! I don't want you to be by yourself! Can he come back??

Lea: Maybe a friend could come over?

Aime: I guess. I'll figure it out.

Emma: Maybe a friend could take the kids for a few hours so you can process?

Lea: I have an excuse to come see you. I'm thinking some restful spa time after your surgery!!

Aime: Good idea! I'll be fine. I just need to work out the logistics. It's very common. People go through this every day.

Lea: It is very common. My neighbor Elizabeth went through it a few years ago. She's totally fine. You are tough. You'll breeze through it.

Aime: Of course ☺

Emma: Definitely!!

I tried to but on a brave face for them and for me. But I was completely shell-shocked. The upbeat tone and "we can beat this" attitude from my sisters helped, so I gathered myself and started driving out of the parking lot.

It was moments like that when I felt the distance between my family and me most acutely. Another woman might be able to just pick up the kids and drive to her sister's house and collapse. Or her mother's. Or her brother's. Or her childhood friend's. But I couldn't. And I knew it was one of the risks we were taking when we made the choice to move to California. When we had made the final decision three years earlier, I called my mom and told her first.

She let out a breath, "You're really going to do it. Well, okay." I was surprised at the time by her reaction. Either way I didn't live in Nashville where she, Dad, and two of my other siblings did, and either way it was a flight to see each other. But somehow she knew it would be different. Farther. A bigger separation.

"It's fine, Mom," I assured her, "It won't be that different than the way it is now, and it won't be forever." It was like she knew somehow. Like she knew that it wasn't going to be fine for me to be so far away.

When she got sick, I felt I was marooned on the other side of the world. I flew back on my own as much as I could, and although my sister Lea bore the brunt of the caretaking, somehow I managed to be there for the big stuff: after the brain surgery when we set up the downstairs bedroom for her, when she was readmitted into the hospital and the doctor told me she wouldn't be going home, and then again in that last move into Intensive Care. It was the downward spiral of increasingly bad news, what the doctors called the "piling on," and I saw it as our lives changing irrevocably with each new development until she ultimately passed away.

Ever since then I had been looking for an out, a way to get back to Boston at least, but it never seemed like the right time. After spending the time to move and get settled into the area, Scott was reluctant to give up the easy access to the biggest tech market in the world. There was too much going on. It was like being trapped in a casino at the blackjack table. We were up a little, and we couldn't leave. We could go on a streak at any moment or we could lose hand after hand.

Scott called back when I was just two minutes down the road. I pulled over, knowing I couldn't concentrate on the road anymore.

The picture is etched clearly in my brain. I pulled over on Alpine Road in Portola Valley under the shade of a tree and struggled to get the words out to Scott. *I have cancer.* I couldn't say it, so I whispered, "It was positive."

It seemed so cruel, the timing of it. I was just starting to think of moving forward in a world without my mother. I was starting to move past the trauma of all that time spent in hospitals watching the life drain out of her. Then just one year and two months after I had said my last words to her, I faced my own diagnosis, my own mortality. But in this case I was on the other side of the country from my family, my husband worked insane hours trying to build his business, and my children still needed me to be present every day in their lives. I was on my own, and I couldn't see how I was going to be able to manage it.

I knew they had caught it early, and I knew there had been great strides made in breast cancer treatment, but I also knew that sometimes when they say your mother should have some good time left to live and wheel her away for brain surgery, she comes back and wakes up talking like a little girl. They said even then she should recover and have eighteen months to live. Three months later she was gone. They say everything will be fine, but I know better than most that sometimes it isn't. It's not fine to watch your beautiful, vibrant, active mother wither away and die in a matter of weeks without ever being able to have a coherent conversation. No last good-byes, no more chances to say that I loved her.

I clutched my phone against my cheek now wet with my tears and barely made my words clear to Scott. How was I going to tell the kids? I had to pick them up from school right then. I couldn't even comprehend what was in front of me. Surgery. Definitely radiation, maybe chemo? How were we going to do this? Who would take care of the children?

He responded in his typically measured way, his strong voice clear across the line, asking a lot of questions, gathering the information, trying to keep things calm and under control. He let me cry and offered his silent strength to steady me. It was his way. Scott lived in a concrete realm. He was a no-nonsense, just-the-facts kind of guy. We comple-mented each other that way. I pulled emotions out of him, and he grounded me in reality when I got off track. I depended on him for that.

I managed one more clear sentence through my tears. "Please come home now."

"Okay. I've already missed the last flight today, but I'll wait at the airport if I have to for the early one tomorrow. I'll be home soon. We'll figure this out."

CHAPTER 2

Ripping Off the Band-Aid

SOMEHOW I PULLED myself together and picked up the kids without incident. One thing almost every mom has had the opportunity to experience is being grateful for children's level of self-absorption when there is something you need to keep from them. I got them home and sat them down with some sort of dinner I pulled together, then I plopped onto the couch with my laptop, desperately seeking information.

The first searches were predictably survival rates for different types and stages. It ranged from 80 to 95 percent. I quickly determined that at this point I had more questions than answers, so I wouldn't be able to glean anything definitive from Google. The next search was simply, "How to tell your kids you have breast cancer."

I happened onto a helpful site with an article on this very issue, the gist of which was: Kids are smart. They know when something is up. Their imaginations will fill in the blanks of what you don't tell them, and their worries might actually be worse than the truth. So tell them the truth, and tell them right away.

I took the advice literally. I had received my marching orders, and I didn't want to spend any more time worrying about it. I told myself it would be like ripping off a Band-Aid—better to do it quickly. Catherine was still at the dinner table, so I sat down across from her. At eleven years old, she was just at that in-between stage of pulling away from me while still depending on me for so many things.

"Hi, Sweetie. I need to talk to you about something."

She looked up at me questioningly.

"So you know that test they took this week at the hospital? Well, what they were checking for was cancer in my breast, and it turns out that I do have it."

Her eyes went wide and I knew she thought of Noni, my mother, whom she had felt very close to.

I took a breath and went on, "But the good news is, it's just a teeny tiny spot, and I just have to do what the doctors tell me to do and I'll be fine."

"So they can get rid of it?" she asked a little hesitantly.

"They do this all the time, and they caught this very early, so that's good." I replied with more confidence than I felt.

"Ok." She looked back down at her phone, visibly relieved.

"Ok," I replied, a little less willing to let it go than she was. "If you want to talk about it or have any questions about anything, just let me know."

"No, I'm good," she said convincingly, looking back up at me and nodding her head.

I pushed up from the table and felt lighter right away. Well that was easy, I thought.

I found Wesley settling into his bed with his iPad. "Hey, Bud. I have something I need to talk to you about."

"Ok," he answered, looking up.

I faltered slightly as I looked into his deep brown eyes, his hair still wet from his shower as he snuggled up on the bottom bunk of his bed with his treasured Lamby slung over his shoulder. He was well past eight years old but still had the habit of carrying his now grayed with age baby stuffy around the house with him. He absentmindedly ran Lamby's torn and ragged ears through his fingers.

I repeated what I had said to Catherine, but Wesley, typical to form, had more questions about it, and the exchange went off like rapid fire.

"So isn't cancer what Noni had?"

"It is, but hers was different because it was in her brain, and by the time the doctors found it, it had gotten too big for them to get it all out. Mine is very small, and the doctors know exactly what they need to do to get rid of it."

"So are they going to have to cut into you to get it out?"

"They are, and it's called surgery. They're very good at it and they will give me medicine so I don't feel it when they do that."

"Oh, that's good. What does it look like?"

"That's a good question, I'm not sure exactly. They called it a little cluster of calcifications, so I would imagine it is white."

"Oh, I thought it would be green or yellow. When are they going to do that?"

"Have my surgery? I still need to find out a lot more information, so I think they're going to take some more tests, and I'll talk to more doctors, and then we'll all decide together. Do you want me to let you know when all of that happens?" I looked carefully at Wesley. He was kicking his feet up onto the bottom of the top bunk and twisting himself in the covers while his fingers continued to work the ears and head of his Lamby.

"Yeah. I want to know every time you go to the doctor and what they say," he said, and then I got it. He was taking a role, and by taking a role he could maintain some semblance of control over the situation.

"You got it, buddy." I ruffled his hair. "I will tell you exactly what is going on."

We spent some cozy time together then and went through his normal bedtime routine. I marveled that while I was so worried about the kids and their reactions to this news, it was they who made me feel better about this whole situation. Life was going on. I had been dealt a blow, but in this moment, I had this treasure, this blissful moment in time with my son.

I turned out the light and whispered good night and Wesley responded, "Mama?"

"Hmm?"

"I just wish you didn't get cancer. I wish it didn't even exist."

"I know, babe. Me too."

Scott got home the next morning and things eased back into a somewhat normal routine. There is no manual for handling news like this. Scott looked at me that night in frustration. "I don't know what to do except to do as many normal things as possible and deal with what we can."

I didn't know what to do either. I didn't know what I needed. We were stunned and paralyzed with helplessness. I went through the motions of the day, but I was living with this heavy pressure of knowing that things were about to change drastically. So I anchored myself with tasks. I got the name of the most highly recommended breast surgeon from my general doctor and quickly set up an initial appointment.

I also received a call from the biopsy surgeon, who, being more used to giving this sort of information than my general doctor had been, was prepared to spend some time with me on the phone. She had gathered more information by then as the pathology reports were more conclusive, so she had a clearer picture of what was going on. It wasn't all good news. She rattled off terms that, while familiar now, seemed like another language at the time.

"So what you have is Invasive Ductal Carcinoma. It's the most common type of breast cancer and highly treatable. You do have a quickly growing type, which is concerning, and that combined with your age is going to encourage aggressive treatment. But the best thing we can see is that your tumor is hormone receptive, which means that it is highly treatable by hormone therapy."

I was trying to digest the information, asking a lot of questions and trying to sort through the answers in my head.

"So do you have a surgeon?" she asked. I told her who my doctor had recommended, and she replied, "That's wonderful. He is who I would have recommended. You will be in great hands. I'm going to give you my cell phone number. Please call me with any questions you have or if you need anything. You're going to get through this."

I had had my chart read once by a well-known and respected astrologist in San Francisco. She ascribed to the belief that our souls come to Earth many times, maybe hundreds or even thousands. Each time we reincarnate into human form, our soul charts a plan, a map of sorts, full of lessons we must learn and things that will happen around us. It's as if we are agreeing to take part in an intricate dance, and while we agree to the form it will take and even the very steps, the passion that we bring to it and the skill we achieve in performing it are up to us.

While my own beliefs had fallen hook, line, and sinker in with those traditional family values and Southern crosses under which I was raised, something about her words had affected me in such a way that even when I heard them the first time, I knew it was something true. It was as if my soul had always known this and she was just reminding my waking self.

As soon as I was alone again with Scott and the kids back to work and school, I locked myself in the bathroom and escaped into a private sanctuary. I let the hot water pour over me in the shower, and my defense shields began to come down. Under all the shock and panic, I felt rage. Suddenly it all hit at once, and I let out the scream I had been holding in for days. I furiously hit the shower wall with the flesh on the side of my fist and gritted my teeth. "It is not time yet, do you hear me? It is not time! I am not finished here. Do you hear me?" I yelled into the air. I yelled at God. At my soul. At the angels. At my mother. At anyone who could hear me.

I seethed and fought against the way that this could turn. I could not imagine my plan that my soul had agreed to could include my leaving my children anytime soon. I've had to deal with some pretty rotten things in my life, and a lot of really beautiful things, too, and I was figuring it all out. But this was too much. This could not be the way it would end. "Not here, not now. This is not happening, I will not allow it!" I screamed.

Finally I collapsed on the floor of the shower in tears.

I felt as if my soul looked on with a patient passivity, with the perspective of knowing the full courses of so many lives. "We'll see," I heard her say in the same voice I heard come out of my own mouth so often when the kids whined about something I didn't really want them to get or do. But I knew that sometimes I let the children have their way. Sometimes it was to teach them something, and sometimes it was because it just didn't matter all that much.

I lay there for a long time, letting the water run over me, and eventually I felt the comfort that whomever I had called to was trying to give me, and I knew I wasn't really alone.

CHAPTER 3

❦

One is Silver and the Other Gold

THE NEXT DAY I was standing in line for pickup at the kid's school. I liked to walk in sometimes instead of waiting in the long car line. It was a way to say hello to the other moms, and the kids always appreciated getting out of the line early. It was another beautiful sunny day, everyone chatting and greeting one another. As I walked into school, I felt the heavy burden of a secret. Each time I saw a smiling face and smiled in return, I wondered behind my mask who I could tell and how I would tell them. I had no idea what lay ahead for me and how it would change my life. Every move I made seemed strange and either totally unnecessary or gravely important.

I was reminded once again that through all my efforts over the past couple of years to get to know people and become a part of the community, the truth was that I was new there. There was no one there I had known for more than two years. There were none of the life-long battle-tested friendships that I knew I could depend on.

I searched through the mass of plaid skirts and navy pants and sweaters for Catherine's blond curls and Wesley's brown moppy hair when Lauren came up and asked me how everything had gone.

I shook my head.

"Shit," she whispered, her pale blue eyes widening. "What are you going to do?"

I shrugged, trying to be brave. What could I do? "Just deal with it."

She hugged me. Catherine had spied me and come over. I waited for Wesley to come out of the line while Lauren's daughter tugged her away toward our friend Shelley. Lauren shook her head, her glossy red hair swinging around her shoulders and said, "Carry on" with a sympathetic smile.

Shelley waved to both of us in greeting but not before I caught a puzzled look. She had seen something pass between Lauren and me but had been too far to hear the words.

"I've just been working on the benefit. Are you all in for a table together? You, us, Jackie and Chris? Who else?"

I pushed away the thoughts clawing at me, relieved by the momentary distraction. "We're in. I talked to Elizabeth Hubbard about joining us, so let's add them as well. How's everything coming?" I looked up at her, craning my neck a bit as she towered over me in her heels.

She must have been six feet tall and habitually wore heels to accentuate her height even further. Her sleek blonde hair was perfectly straightened without a single stray, and her electric blue eyes were lined with a smudge of eyeliner to make them pop as if the bright blue color itself were not enough to make you notice. She always had the look of having just come from an outdoor lunch with one of the Silicon Valley heavyweights. The scent of money seemed to hang around her, and the careful way she put together her words made it perpetually seem as if she had just made a new multi-million-dollar real estate deal she couldn't tell anyone about yet.

"Great," she replied. "We have some new items to add for the live auction. I think the catalog is filling in nicely. I'll get the details in to Dan, and then you will be able to write them up."

Crap. Catalog writing. I had committed to write the auction item descriptions along with a "team" of others, and so far no one else had been wrangled to join. "Yes, I'd love to be able to knock those out quickly," I said. Hopefully I could get a good chunk done before the surgery and then someone else could step up. Just add it to the list.

Lauren was looking back and forth between us, the undercurrents palpable in the air. "Okay, well, we're in too! I've got to go get Emily, but let me know." She escaped quickly.

Shelley looked down at her phone as it lit up with a notification. "It's Jackie," she said with a grin. "I texted her some pics of the kids from the field trip. Have you talked to her?"

I shook my head, tucking my windblown hair behind my ear and smoothing it out, "Not since she's been away. I've seen the photos on Facebook, though. It looks like she's having a beautiful trip."

"She looks radiant. A week in the Spanish Riviera will do that to a lady." Shelley widened her eyes and sighed.

"I know, sign me up for that work trip," I said. Jackie worked her tail off as a director for a major consulting firm, and I knew that she deserved to add a few vacation days to her client meetings overseas, but I couldn't help but be envious of her jet set lifestyle.

"When is she coming back again?" I asked.

"Saturday, I think. Not soon enough, I miss her. We haven't had a catch-up in almost a month." She smiled and then gave a little pout.

One thing Shelley and I had always had in common was how much we loved Jackie.

"I know, she's been traveling so much for work, our relationship has been reduced to mostly texts lately."

"I count on her to keep me organized with what is going on at school," Shelley admitted, "I missed Eucharist this past Thursday because she didn't remind me. I honestly don't know what I would do without her."

"Mama," Wesley pulled on my arm impatiently.

"I've got to run, too," I said, knowing she would wonder what happened between Lauren and me. I would have to tell her later.

We waved and split off. I patted Wesley's back between his shoulder blades that jut out like little wings and Catherine stood up from sitting on her rolling backpack. "Finally!" she said. "You guys were talking forever!"

"Mom talk," I said, reaching out with my other arm and holding her while I kissed her on the crown of her head, inhaling her scent like perfume. Salt, musk, coconut…she always smelled like she'd been at the beach all day.

CHAPTER 4

❧

Game On

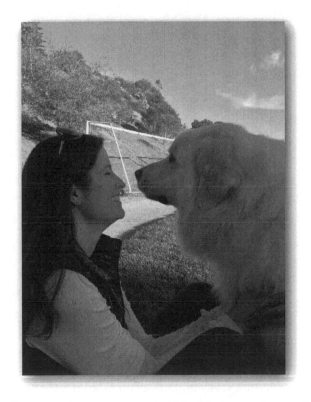

I WOKE ON Monday morning to a text Jackie had sent the night before:

Jackie: Hey girl! Got home from Spain late last night. Amazing trip with hubby! Been thinking of you and hope you are feeling okay. Anxious to hear about med update. Xoxo

Aime: Hi! Looked like you had a beautiful trip. I'm so glad! It was fun to see pics on fb.

I took a deep breath. I didn't want to sit on the news any longer. It was just so hard to talk about it, to say the words out loud over and over. I had always found communication much easier by writing than speaking because I had a better understanding of how my words appeared when I saw them on paper, or at least on my phone. And I supposed it also gave me a layer of protection and fed my conscious or unconscious need for a buffer from other people's thoughts, emotions, and opinions.

Aime: So it turns out it was bad news for me. I've got a struggle ahead. Xo
Jackie: Oh no! My dear friend I'm sorry!!! Any way I could take you to dinner tonight? We might need a glass of wine for this one. Or are you better with coffee?
Aime: Red wine in moderation is on the approved list ☺ tonight Catherine has her Holy Cross interview—maybe the morning.
Jackie: Let's do coffee tomorrow morning. Is that okay? Xoxoxo
Aime: Perfect.

The parking gods were smiling on me as I found a spot right in front of the Sharon Heights Starbucks. I rushed in, found my spot in line, and glanced around for Jackie. It was the usual mix of paunchy, silver-haired venture capitalists having meetings implicitly stated as casual but that could have involved buying or selling any number of companies blended with soccer moms grabbing that extra boost of morning caffeine and donning Lululemon outfits designed both for exercise and as socially acceptable substitutes for pajamas, and programmers or engineers trying to find a spot near but removed from Stanford. The latter were most easily spotted by their lithe frames, wire glasses, rumpled clothes, and high-powered laptops they ducked their heads behind.

I was running a little behind, so when I got there Jackie was already waiting with my drink and a sandwich. As I walked to meet her, I inhaled the scent of coffee, caramel, and mocha that every Starbucks somehow seems to share.

"Hi!" she greeted me with her typical bright smile, but I saw the concern in the slight creases of her eyes. She was dressed to the nines, as always, with her perfect light brown hair with blonde highlights cropped neatly into a bob under her chin and flawless nails and makeup. It was always fun to see her before work because I could tell by the way she dressed what kind of day she had lined up. Today was obviously client meetings evidenced by her chunky pearls and bouclé jacket with heels. She pulled me over to the table she had secured with her bag and our breakfast.

Jackie was a couple of inches shorter than me, and we shared the tendency toward a curvy figure, which, while normal by any standard, we commiserated about nevertheless, especially when we compared ourselves to the impossibly tall and thin pair of Shelley and Lauren.

"Okay, so eat. You need to keep up your strength. And tell me everything," she said, her mothering instincts naturally suggesting that comfort food was a necessary accompaniment to a conversation about cancer.

I picked at the sandwich and let it all pour out. I cried. Right there in Starbucks. My regular Starbucks. Not the ugly cry, but tears flowed steadily like a cup that's been filled just the slightest bit too much.

"I know it's highly treatable. There's no mystery here. They know just what to do, and I think I would be okay about it all if it wasn't for Mom."

"I know," she nodded and tears filled her eyes. It had only been the year before we had sat in this very place while she held my hands as I worried about my mother. "You're having a very challenging year. But you know what? You are one of the strongest, wisest women I know, and if anyone can get through this, it's you. God doesn't give us more than we can handle, but Lord, he must think a lot of you." Her green eyes twinkled with dampness.

I let out a breathy laugh through my tears, and she joined me with her best girlfriend chuckle.

"I'd like to have a conversation with God about all of this. I think my strength might have been oversold."

"No. You've got this. And you don't have to do it alone, either. I want you to know that you have support. You have us—your friends, and me, and Chris. We will all be here for you, and we will figure this out." We finished up our drinks, and the time grew later into the morning.

"Ok, my dear. So now let me know what I can do. I know the rest of the class moms are going to want to know about this and are going to want to help. So when you decide you are ready, I will send out an email to the class moms. In the meantime, think about what your needs might be. I know this isn't easy for you and that you don't like to ask for help, but remember that people are going to want something to do. So think of everything—playdates, meals, rides to the hospital, company for appointments, whatever—and then leave it all to me."

"Honestly, I don't know right now, but I will think about it. I'll come up with some kind of list, but I think we'll need to wait and see how things go. Right now I just have the surgery planned and I think we have to go from there to see what happens after."

"Okay, well you just let me know. Love you." She gave me a big squeeze and kissed my cheek. She looked into my eyes with her brightest smile. "You are a beautiful, strong and vivacious woman who will handle this all with grace. I'm here for you, and so is Chris."

I spent the next few days developing an aggressive healing strategy and exploring all my options, from reiki and acupuncture to naturopaths. I kept busy with appointments of all kinds. First came the appointment with Dr. D. Scott planned to meet me for the afternoon appointment, so I drove to Stanford by myself. Getting to Stanford took about twenty-five minutes from our house, but once on campus the maze of construction and multiple winding roads and miles of buildings took me another twenty minutes to navigate through. I was directed to a parking garage and then instructed to take a shuttle to the cancer center. Being unable or unwilling to say "Cancer Center" out loud, I called it by the building name, Blake Wilbur. When I got off the shuttle, a helpful worker asked the address I was looking for, and when I told her, she smiled and pointed me toward another building. I walked past a valet parking station and noted the prices, thinking there would be days that it would be worth it.

Stanford is set up like so many other structures in California with a series of outdoor walkways leading between smaller buildings as the weather rarely requires a need for cover. I walked between two massive concrete planters with trees in them and through a double set of automatic glass doors that opened with a quiet whoosh as I approached. The women's center was marked clearly and I found myself standing in line to announce myself in a pleasant lounge behind a sign encouraging patients to "wait here in respect of others' privacy" several feet back from the reception desk.

I checked in and waited, all the while looking around at the other patients. I couldn't help it. I wanted to see who else was dealing with the same thing I was. There were probably only four or five other patients, none of them close to my age. I guessed they were sixty and older. They each had someone with them—a spouse, friend, family member, or sometimes a nurse. I also noticed varied stages of hair, hats, and potential wigs. It was all new to me.

Scott rushed into the lounge and spotted me. He sat down with a sigh. "That parking garage is a nightmare."

"I know, I just got here myself." I checked the time on my phone. It had only been a couple of minutes, and we were right on time for the appointment.

We were called back, and after the nurse checked my vitals and I changed into a medical gown, a knock on the exam room door announced the presence of Dr. D. He entered the room and intro-duced himself to both of us. He was exactly how I hoped he would be. Older than me, but not by too much, he had a calm, quiet, and understated demeanor. His clothes and hair were conservative and slightly rumpled, and his eyes seemed a little tired behind his wire-rimmed glasses.

"It's nice to meet you," he said, shaking my hand, "although I wish we could have met somewhere better like the Apple store instead of being here for this." He smiled, his sympathy seeming genuine. I imag-ined he'd seen a lot of tears in his line of work.

He got down to business and went through my chart and com-pleted an exam. Then he sat down while I wrapped the gown around myself and sat up straight on the table.

He looked at Scott and me and said, "First I'm going to order an MRI for both breasts so we have a very clear picture of anything that is going on. Just be forewarned, the MRIs are very sensitive. They pick up absolutely everything, so don't be surprised if something shows up. We just want to be very thorough in this case and if anything at all shows up, we're going to check it out. Then we're going to need to do the surgery within the next two to three weeks. Right now we still don't have all the information we need to determine your total treatment, but I would think of it as a nine-month process. If it turns out to be less, that's great. It really depends on how the pathology comes back from the surgery whether or not chemotherapy will be recommended. At this point it's too early to know for sure. You're going to go through a lot of ups and downs in the next few months, so I would try to stay as steady as you can. And plan something nice to look forward to at the end of all this. Maybe a nice trip."

Scott had been taking notes, uncomfortably bent over a spiral notebook resting on his knee and scrawling words out with his left hand. He looked up and smiled at me. "We can do that," he nodded. It seemed to be the first good thing he had heard in weeks.

"As far as the actual surgery goes," Dr. D went on, "the options would be a lumpectomy or a mastectomy, and some women opt for a double mastectomy. There are various theories and suggestions, but for you I would be comfortable with whatever you choose. A lumpectomy would be sufficient for now but would need to be followed by radiation. If you do a mastectomy, then you would not need to follow with radiation, but whether or not you do chemotherapy is determined based on the pathology and lymph node involvement, so a mastectomy wouldn't preclude chemotherapy. The reason most people do the double mastectomy is because of the high risk of cancer appearing in the second breast and also for cosmetic purposes."

He paused to let the information sink in. "You can take a little time to think about it. We'll have one more appointment before the surgery and you can make the call then."

To keep or not to keep my breasts. That was the question. It would take some time for me to sort that one out. I didn't feel particularly attached to them, but there was something awful about the prospect of cutting off part of my body. I assumed the surgery would be a bear, although I hadn't looked into it much yet. My ambivalent relationship to my breasts began when they started growing when I was just twelve. They started growing and didn't quit until they landed in a place that for years I squeezed into a 36C, but really I was a solid D cup, if not a DD. It was a lot for my frame to carry, and before all you beautifully small and perky-breasted women judge me for taking for granted my generous cup size, I would encourage you to try to imagine going through junior high with boobs that big. By the time I finished high school I called them the bane of my existence. I was so jealous of my sister Lea's lithe runner's body.

Now that they actually did threaten my existence I knew painfully well how terrible it was to hate a part of my own body. I did start to appreciate them more when I was able to enjoy the miracle of breastfeeding with Catherine and Wesley, and thankfully after that process they had thinned out to a more acceptable shape, I thought. Then by the time I moved to California I was shocked to be asked by more than one person if they were real. I was happy to point out that I had the matching ass as proof.

But what I really felt more strongly than anything at that point was just, GET IT OUT! I didn't even really care how. Every night when I went to sleep I worried about this cancer that was growing in my body. It seemed that every day that passed while it lived inside me was putting me more and more at risk. I worried about sleeping on my left side. Would it encourage the cells to travel down toward my lymph nodes? What about what I ate? I had researched all the cancer growth-promoting foods and cancer-fighting foods and was trying desperately to change my diet. I was juicing like a green monster, trying to flood my body with healthy vitamins. I would do whatever they told me would work. I would cut off my breasts without a second thought if they told me to, but they were leaving it up to me and that was a decision I was too overwhelmed to make.

I had gotten quiet, so Dr. D started talking to Scott. "So how are things at home? Do you think you have the support you will need? Do you have family around?"

Scott shook his head and cleared his throat. "No, we just moved out here a couple of years ago, and all of our family is back East, but we're looking into hiring some help now, and a lot of our friends from the kids' school have offered to help out. I think we'll be okay."

"We have resources here at the hospital if you need them. Support groups, informational classes, there are all kinds of things in here." He handed Scott a glossy folder stuffed full of papers and information. "There is also this great program called Bay Area Cancer Connections in Palo Alto." He looked back at me, "You should look into them. Sometimes it really helps to have a group of people to fall back on. Or just someone to talk to that understands."

He stood and looked at us both. "It's not easy, what you're going through. It seems particularly hard for people your age, at this stage in your life. You should know that there are people out there who can help you."

"Thanks," Scott and I both mumbled. It was a lot to digest. Dr. D gave us our next steps, and Scott wrote everything out. Then we said our good-byes. Dr. D closed the door behind him, and I looked at Scott. He stood up and put his arm around me, and I cried softly into his chest.

CHAPTER 5

Going Public

THE NEXT ORDER of business was figuring out exactly what kind of help and support I would be needing. It was more complicated than one would think. It was hard to quantify everything that I did during the course of a day or a week or a month because it consisted of so many little things, some of which were nonessential, but many of which were critical to the feeding, education, and clothing of my family.

Jackie, Shelley, and Lauren had all been gently prodding to see what I needed, but it took me a while just to process all of this life-changing information and to get organized enough to be able to give them any kind of a clear list.

Shelley finally tracked me down and got me to join her for a quick Starbucks stop one afternoon. I walked in to join her and paused as an elderly man held the door open for his wife, who was taking careful steps with a cane. My heart ached watching them, two wispy white-haired heads bent close together with hands intertwined. I had not been able to see my parents reach that stage together, and I wondered, would our children see Scott and me that way? I was doubtful. I knew I had a good chance of surviving this breast cancer, but the higher risk of cancer I might be left with and the toll all of the treatment might take on my body seemed to make my own chances of reaching that age slim.

Shelley waved at me and motioned for me to join her a few people ahead in line. No matter how many times I had been in there, I was still amused by the scene when I entered this tiny snapshot of Silicon

Valley. I felt as if I were pretending to belong. Shelley, however, was right in her element. This was her crowd.

We sat down outside in a pair of oversized lounge chairs with well-worn cushions that were pushed back under an ample awning against the exterior windows.

"How are you?" Shelley asked, pushing her straightened blond hair back with her sunglasses.

I hesitated. It was an automatic greeting, but I couldn't answer honestly any more.

"I'm fine. Just busy trying to get things squared away." I fumbled with the wrapper of the straw. The paper had gotten wet, so I had to peel it away before I punched the straw through the plastic lid of my green tea lemonade.

"I'm sure. We're all anxious to find a way to help you." She nodded as she passed a napkin over to my side of the table.

"I know, it's just hard to know what to ask for. There are so many random and different things that I do, and I don't know what my limitations will be exactly. I feel like I'm preparing for a big snow storm or a long journey, only I don't know exactly how long I'll be gone or where I'm going." I shook my head.

Shelley smiled. "That's beautifully put. I can imagine how difficult this must be for you. I know you're working hard to get your benefit tasks done, and I'm trying to take that off your plate. I just want to find another way to take some of your burden away. I know people have talked about doing meals..." She let her words trail off for a moment before continuing on, "I just want you to know that I want to be there for you very much, but I'm a terrible cook. I hope I can find some other way to help."

I laughed. "I know, I always hesitate to sign up to bring people meals myself. Don't worry about that at all. It's not my biggest concern. Scott's parents didn't know what to do, so they just sent us a huge gift certificate for Munchery. That should keep us fed for awhile."

"Oh, what's Munchery?"

"It's this great app where you can order fresh farm to table food cooked by local chefs and delivered to your door." I pulled up the app and showed it to her, scrolling through the beautiful photos of dinners available for that night.

"Oh, I need that too!" Shelley perked up considerably. "It would limit the number of times I have to call Town for takeout on my way home."

"It's a huge time saver. The only problem is the kids don't love it. They'll take pasta or corn dogs any day over tofu sloppy joes and pan-crusted snapper. But if all else fails, there's always peanut butter and jelly. The dinner of champions."

Over the next few days trouble began to stir in the benefit committee, of which all of us—with the exception of Jackie, who was too busy and too smart to get involved—were a part. I had missed a meeting in which Lauren, frustrated by the amount of work that was being piled on her as the new person, blew up and quit. Shelley, with skills acquired from years of dealing with the most difficult real estate clients imaginable, tried in vain to smooth things over, but after Lauren stormed out the committee turned to her pressuring Shelley to get me to step in for Lauren. Shelley tried to dismiss me as an option, saying that I was too busy with other things, but my name kept coming up as the only alternative until Shelley uncharacteristically lost her cool and suggested that I had some personal issues going on and for them to leave me alone.

Of course at that point I heard immediately from the co-chair in an email asking me if I was also quitting. I wasn't completely clear about what had happened, but I knew I didn't want to take on an even bigger role in something that I cared less and less about each day, so I thought I should just tell the committee what was going on. Shelley disagreed, insisting that my business was my own and they didn't deserve an excuse, and she didn't want to tell them. So I was left to just finish my work and quietly, but gladly, bow out of the committee.

Since I had some time to absorb the situation, I could see that what I really was sensitive about was not people knowing what was going on with me but doing the actual telling myself. People in my life would have to know eventually. I would lose my hair, not show up for things. It wasn't something I could or needed to keep a secret. I didn't know why Shelley felt so strongly about keeping the news private, but I didn't really agree with her. I just needed a point person. I needed someone to spread the news so people would know why I needed to step back a little and cut me some slack. Maybe that was one of the things I really needed to learn. I shouldn't have had to get cancer to quit worrying about making everyone else happy. Because that was a no-win game.

Then, just a few days later, I officially went public. Through Jackie.

From: Bowen, Jackie
Sent: Friday, February 28, 2014 1:18 PM
To: 2nd Grade moms
Subject: please read

Dear 2nd grade moms,

We don't always get the chance to reflect on how blessed our lives are. Suddenly we can be faced with a significant challenge to overcome—one which we shouldn't and can't face alone.
It's with that in mind I share some news about our sweet Aime Card. She has been diagnosed with stage 2 breast

cancer and will be undergoing surgery on March 5th. Aime will be going through radiation and potentially chemotherapy following the surgery. Although long term prognosis is good, it's scary and I know she would love your prayers during this time. I'm sure you can appreciate the sensitivity and privacy Aime and her family need during this time, but we also wanted to have the community come together and support them as well. Dropping a line or a voicemail would warm her heart and I know bring a smile to her face, as she's not prepared to talk about it yet.

As such, I'll be reaching out to help coordinate various things over the next few months like dinners, after-school pickup and playdates, which would be of help to Aime.

Blessings and many thanks,
Jackie

I was flooded that morning with beautiful notes from the other parents in the class either sent directly to me or to Jackie, who forwarded along their sympathy and willingness to help in any way. But there were a couple of panicked messages peppering me with demands for details and plans and, "Oh my God, what are you going to do? What about the kids? Please call me as soon as you can!" Although I understood the sentiment, the tone of those messages and the tax on me was huge in a time I could least afford to handle it. It pained me, and I distanced myself from these people. I answered back by text or email that I was still finding out the details but doing well and would keep them posted. It was all I could do. I knew they meant well, but their panic was feeding my own, and I would still be left with cancer when they moved on to the next mini-crisis. To me this wasn't a mini-crisis; this was life or death.

It was also time to share the news with Catherine and Wesley's teachers and Rachael, the head of school, so I sent out an email.

From: Aime Card
Subject: Family Update

Hello Rachael, Brenda and Matthew,

I just wanted to give you an update about something that is going on in our family. I have recently been diagnosed with breast cancer. We are in the middle of setting up treatment options and plans to move forward, but it will almost certainly impact Catherine and Wesley in some fashion. They are aware of what's going on and are familiar with the proper terms (no euphemisms here), and they seem okay with it at this point. We have been careful to stay optimistic and positive.

The first step will be for me to have surgery, which will most likely take place within the next three weeks. I won't be able to drive for at least two weeks and possibly more depending on the option for surgery that we choose, so my father will be staying with us and driving for the kids.

Please feel free to share this with whomever you feel needs to know, but if you could let me know who you do share with, I would appreciate it. I haven't talked to many people about it yet because the news is still pretty tender for me and there are still so many outstanding variables.

Many thanks for your understanding.

Aime

I heard back almost immediately from Catherine's teacher.

From: Brenda Carmichael
Subject: Re: Family Update

Hi Aime,

I am so terribly sorry to hear this scary news. I expect that you must feel overwhelmed with great concern for your family. Thank you for letting me know so I can not only support you but support Catherine as well.

I don't know if you know this, but I also had breast cancer. I am a very happy 15 year survivor this year. I remember well the shock of being diagnosed and having to very quickly come up with a plan to battle it. In my case it included surgery, chemotherapy, and radiation therapy. I know there are different kinds of breast cancer and many successful medical treatments, so I don't know what your specific case is like. I would be more than happy to talk with you if you would like. I found it helpful to talk to women who were going through cancer at the same time as me and to other women who had been through before and survived.

I encourage you to reach out for support as you feel comfortable. I remember that it was important to just go day by day dealing with decisions as they came up, along with keeping my life as normal as possible surrounded by the love of my family. If you think it would be helpful, please tell Catherine that I am also a breast cancer survivor and would be happy to talk to her privately if she would like. This is going to be a challenging journey for all of you. I pray that you will come through it with strength and love of others supporting you all the way.

Much love,
Brenda

Reading her email brought a flood of relief and something to hold onto. She was the first woman I knew personally who had been through breast cancer and survived, not only through the initial crisis but for fifteen long years after. We started a correspondence that gave me a great deal of strength.

The next day we pulled up to our little stucco house tucked between the overgrown agave plants and redwood trees, and we saw a large package at the front door. Catherine and Wesley hopped out of the car, slamming the doors behind them, and ran over to investigate.

"Oh, look!" Catherine said, "It's from Nashville!" She bounced up and down with a big grin. She loved everything in my hometown—barbeque, Papa's big house with the pool, all the old toys Mom had saved, and most especially all her cousins. She once told me that she thought Nashville was her "true home" even though she'd never lived there.

I opened the big box and out fell a bunch of M&Ms and a stack of drawings from my nieces and nephews. Catherine and Wesley went through these quickly and taped them all up on the fridge. I pulled out a small tissue-wrapped package that held a palm-sized brown leather-bound book with gold-lined pages. In gold script was embossed "Marion Alley" on the front corner. I ran my fingers over the letters, remembering my mother's warm hand when I held it last. I opened the book to the first page and saw, "Daily Light for Every Day presented to Mom by Fronda and Rob." Under the inscription Rob had written, "Her children rise up and call her blessed. Prov. 31:28, February 20, 2004."

On the inside of the jacket a pink note was attached with my mother's handwriting, "For the eyes of the Lord range throughout the earth to strengthen those whose hearts are fully committed to him. 2. Chron. 9."

My brother's wife, Fronda, had tucked in a note,

"Aime, we are praying for you and thinking about you and hoping good things. I know you're going to be okay. You are strong and positive. We want to help any way we can—please let us know if you can think of anything. We are sending you Marion's robe, some candy and the devotional we gave Marion when she was first diagnosed. I wish she was here to tell you it's going to be okay. You have her strength, Aime. I love the verse Marion put on the inside of the devotional. Believe it. We love you, Fronda and Rob"

My eyes filled with tears as I pulled the thick white terry cloth robe out of the box. I carried it down to my bedroom and wrapped it around me. It smelled like home. I fell to my knees and sobbed.

CHAPTER 6

❧

Goddess of Wisdom

THE FEAR STARTED creeping more and more steadily into my life. One night I was sitting on the couch, and my left arm started getting numb and tingly. I started seeing black spots and I turned to Scott in a panic, and then it just faded away as easily as it had come. I knew it must have been a minor panic attack, but I also knew that I was going to have to find a better way to deal with the stress of all of this or it would come out sideways.

The acupuncturist I had been seeing recommended for me to call an energy healer. "She's amazing," she said. "A therapist who talked to her told me that she would put her out of business."

I booked a session immediately. I would try anything. Her office was in Fresno, and I didn't have time to make the drive out, so we agreed to speak on the phone. "Location doesn't matter," she had said when she made the appointment. "I'm just happy I can help."

I called at the appropriate time and lay down on my bed as I was instructed to get comfortable, as if for meditation. My meditation spot was my bed, so there I was. I had seen Diane's picture on the website, so I mentally held her image while she spoke. She was probably in her late forties or early fifties and aging very well. She had naturally silver hair that was straight and hung to her shoulders, and beautiful shining eyes.

"So tell me what's going on," she said as she started off the session.

I filled her in on my health issues and said, "I think the biggest thing I am dealing with right now is the fear. I've been having nightmares and panic attacks."

"Yes," she said, "can you explain that a little bit?"

"Well, I guess it's just the obvious. It's the fear that this is it. Fear that I won't make it through."

"Let's take it back a step. So the doctors have explained to you that this is treatable, that it's something that the overwhelming majority of people who deal with survive. So where is your fear coming from?"

"I think this is hitting me harder than it normally would because my mom passed away from cancer last year."

"Uh huh." Diane responded. "So you think the same thing will happen to you?"

"Well, yes, I guess I do. Maybe not right now, but maybe not too long from now. And the real thing is, I'm not so much afraid of dying for myself. It's just that I can't leave the kids. They're too young." A few tears escaped as I confessed to Diane what I thought was the essential truth.

"Yes. Every mother has that fear, and here you've been dealt a serious blow that has placed this fear in the forefront of your mind. How old are your children?"

"They're 8 and 11."

"Okay. Well, let me explain one thing to you right off the bat. Fear is a negative emotion. It can't create anything; it's like a dead end. It doesn't go anywhere. The only thing that can alter the course of things is positive energy. So with the fear you are wasting the opportunity to create positive change. The fear can't do anything negative to you on its own, but it won't allow you to change the course you are on. Whatever you focus on that is greater than your fear is what you receive. So for example with the bad dreams, when you wake up and remember them, just rethink them with a positive ending. Change the story and you'll see that the power of them just goes away."

"And about your children," she continued, "do you think part of your fear there is about not being able to do as much for them?"

"Yes, I know it is. I haven't even been able to come up with a list of how I need help because it is too overwhelming to think about not being able to do these things for them myself."

"But at their ages, they are really able to understand what's going on. Maybe you should talk to them about some extra responsibilities that they can take on. That could serve two purposes. One, to take some of the load off of you and what you are worrying about, and two, it can really make them feel empowered to be able to do something to help the situation."

I nodded and then remembered she couldn't see me. "I think you're right. They do love having little chores and responsibilities around the house, so often I just end up doing things myself to make it faster or get it done the way I want it to be done, but I know I can and need to let that go. Especially now."

"That's right. Even when kids grumble and complain at first, the responsibilities are really good for them in so many ways."

"Huh," I responded, my mind reeling with the possibilities of all that she had said.

"So let's get back to the fear now. Taking the kids out of the equation, where do you think the next level of the fear is?"

"Another thing I'm actively afraid of right now is that I won't wake up from the surgery. I know it's unlikely for that to happen, but it does happen sometimes. And already I know that when something is unlikely to happen, it doesn't mean that it won't. It was unlikely for me to get breast cancer at my age, but I did. It was unlikely for my beautiful, healthy mother to die at her age, but she did."

"Okay, we're going to work on this. So are you comfortable? Let's get started."

She led me through a guided meditation with the intention of bringing me back into myself and the present moment by naming various parts of my body and asking me to relax each one starting with my toes and ending around my shoulders, neck, cheeks, mouth, eyes and forehead.

"Now let's take a minute to drop into your body and just do a check. See if you can let yourself drop into your left breast. Sit there for a minute. What do you feel there?"

I saw red images in my mind, and then I started to feel a prickly sensation that I described to her along with visions of white spiked streaks of light that felt like broken glass. The light seemed to gather in several balls before my eyes of various sizes, resembling the prickly pear seeds I used to find as a child.

I tried to describe the feelings to her and she responded, "So think about that prickly feeling. Does it remind you of anything? Have you felt that before?"

I thought for a moment and then suddenly I was able to clearly relate the feeling, "Yes. It feels like the fear for my children's safety. Just the stress of keeping them alive as babies and toddlers."

"That's right," she said. "Now think about that fear. Did it come from you?"

An image came into my mind of my mother, shaking her hands in worry over something dangerous I was doing.

"No, I think it came from my mom."

"That's right. Whenever an emotion causes a physical sensation in our body it's a clue to us that it came from someone else. So why do you think you took on that fear?"

"I think I needed it. I needed it to feel like I was a good mother." Even as I said it, I sort of laughed at how backwards it sounded. That I would need fear to prove that I loved my children was ludicrous.

"That's right. So do you think you can let that go?"

"Yes," I sighed and readily agreed. I did not need that fear anymore. Being cautious was not the same thing as being afraid, and by then I knew the difference.

"So let's take a moment to let that go. Just let it fall away into Mother Earth where she can take it and recycle it into something different."

I sat quietly for a moment and felt the fear just melting away from my body and dripping down beneath me into the deep brown earth.

"Okay, so let's go back into your breast. Is there anything else there?"

I thought for a moment and then I felt this overwhelming anxiety. I described it to Diane, and she asked me, "So do you remember the last time you felt that feeling?"

"Yes," I knew exactly when. "It was when my mom was sick. It's not the sadness from after she died, but the worry and helpless feelings surrounding her illness. I have tried so hard to heal and process her death, but I really haven't even been able to think about the trauma of just her being sick, and all the planning and the hospital stays and the helpless feeling of being so far away and not being able to do more for her."

"That's right. So do you think you can let that go now?"

"Yes," I agreed and knew that it was time. I let all of those feelings melt away just like I had with the fear for the kids.

"So now. Go into your breast and see what's left there."

I thought for a couple of minutes; it seemed to take longer then. Just when I was about to say I didn't see anything, I felt a profound sadness. I described it to Diane and she asked me if I recognized that feeling.

My heart broke.

"Yes." I said. "It's my baby. The one I lost."

Diane was quiet while I cried for a minute or two.

"It was an early miscarriage. I thought I had moved past it a long time ago, but I guess I've been still holding onto the grief somewhere deep inside."

"Okay," Diane said softly after a minute. "You need to know that separation is only an illusion. There is no separation with love. Unconditional love is eternal."

"Yes, I believe that." I said through my tears.

"So are you ready to let go of that pain?"

"Yes." We sat quietly together while an image came to my mind of a tiny white bundle. I gathered the bundle in my arms and laid it down gently knowing it was safe in the arms of Mother Earth. I cried softly but was surrounded by a deep feeling of peace.

"Good work, Aime."

I said goodbye to Diane and knew that in that one short hour, fear and pain that I had held onto for years had vanished.

CHAPTER 7

❧

Pulp Fiction Moment March

A COUPLE OF nights before my surgery my phone started lighting up with texts from Shelley.

Shelley: I'm having a second glass of wine to deal with benefit stuff ☺ A Pinot in your honor, actually.

Shelley: Well it was the open bottle but the Pinot made me think of you so still very honorable.

Shelley: Are you up for coffee tomorrow?

Aime: Can't tomorrow. Have to meet the surgeon one more time and then pick up Dad.

Shelley: Jees prioirites... Doctors and Dad. I will try not to take it personally. Are you feeling strong?

Aime: Sort of. I had Reiki today and that was nice. Maverick is freaking me out, though. He keeps following me around and he's moping.

Shelley: He feels the anxious energy, maybe. Talk to him. Tell him you need his support and strength and that all is good. Or is that weird? I believe in animal's energy. I still have dreams of my favorite deceased cat. I feel she still comes to comfort me.

Aime: I'm sure she does. I have heard sometimes that animals can try to take on your hurt or sickness, and I keep telling him he doesn't have to do that. I keep telling him we're going to get better at the same time. His breed has one of the best noses too, so he might even smell the cancer. Maybe he'll get better once it's all gone after the surgery.

Shelley: Probably. Keep telling him what you need and for him to keep watching over you and the family. Reminding him of his job might make him feel better.

Shelley: Is he sick?

Aime: He threw up once and he has this sore on his nose that won't heal. Not serious though.

Shelley: ☹ We should give him Reiki.

Aime: I'm trying. I've got to get to bed.

Shelley: Sorry. Hugs and kisses. Have wonderful dreams knowing you are loved by all around you. I am sending positive thoughts to you and Mav.

On the day of my surgery I was told to check in by 6:30 a.m., so Scott and I had to leave in the morning before the kids woke up. Dad had come in the night before in time to share a big steak dinner with us that felt celebratory. He heard us getting ready to leave and came out of the study, still brushing down his hair and wearing his undershirt. He gave me a smile and patted my shoulder. "Good luck, sweetie. It'll all be fine. I've got the kids."

As Scott drove me to the hospital in silence, it reminded me of an early morning drive to the hospital years before in Boston when I was in labor with Catherine. That morning had been so different, but similar in ways. Eleven years earlier, nervous excitement was the predominant feeling, but as we pulled into the surgical center, all I felt were the nerves.

"Prep" is a nice term that the surgical team gives to hours of invasive procedures. It was after 3:00 p.m. before I was greeted by the surgeon. My MRI had turned up three more troubling spots that the team wanted to check out, so in addition to the tissue removal for the site around the tumor, they would remove tissue from and test three other areas as well as my lymph nodes. I had spent hours being injected by radioactive dye, having three wires guided and placed by ultrasound, and waiting. After a while I forgot about my hunger and thirst and maintained a faint empty feeling. I took my first Ativan that day, a drug I came to know well in the following months. It calmed my nerves and settled my stomach, allowing me to sit back and watch impassively as the world marched by. Unfortunately I had taken it at 7:00 a.m. in the first waiting room, so by the time the anesthesiologist came in at 3:00 p.m. to introduce himself and assess me, it was starting to wear off.

He laughed, "Don't worry. I'll get you hooked up soon. You won't feel a thing."

Scott had stayed in the various waiting rooms all day, fielding calls and emails and passing updates to our families and to Jackie, who had been put in charge of updating the others. We finally sat together as the team made the final preparations. Scott's eyes were tired and strained, but he sat by me with a steadfast solidity that always reassured me. That was the thing about him; he always made me feel safe.

He had the look of a former athlete that had gone a little soft. He was the first to poke fun at his attempts to remain in shape, but his stressful job and long hours never allowed it. When we met, he was in business school at Tuck in New Hampshire. I think he chose it over MIT because of its proximity to the ski resorts because he skied fifty days that spring. Once I went with him, and while I was just a beginner following the trail, he tried to impress me by jumping over the rocks ahead of me. Instead I was impressed by the size of his massive yard sale when he fell right in front of me—arms, legs, skis, and poles flying in every direction. We laughed for days at that one.

He had worked for years on Wall Street to earn what he considered the break of business school. Wall Street for analysts was considerably less scandalous and glamorous than the papers would have you believe. He worked like a dog for four years straight, regularly pulling all-nighters in the office and crunching numbers repeatedly for months on end. He burned out at the end and was feeling more like a normal person when we met after a year at school, but interviews started that spring, and he went right back into banking. Ever since then he'd been slogging his way through it climbing the ladder, his only concession being that he got to stay in Boston, the town he loved. Until we moved to California. And now this.

"Can you hold my hand?" I asked, craving his solid touch. He stretched out his hand gingerly as if he were afraid I might break.

"It's going to be fine," he assured me in his soft deep voice that spread over me like a balm.

"How long can he stay with me?" I asked the anesthesiologist, and I watched his face change from cheerful to sympathetic.

"We're going to walk down the hall now, and he can say good-bye just outside the room. You'll be asleep within seconds, don't worry. Okay, ready?" he gestured to the team and they moved and adjusted an assortment of medical equipment in a well-choreographed dance and wheeled me in my bed toward the surgical room.

"Okay, time to say good-bye now." The anesthesiologist smiled.

"Good luck," Scott whispered as he kissed my forehead, "I'll be right outside."

His hand left mine and I was whisked away. An oxygen mask was placed over my face and I heard, "Ok, Aime, just take a few deep breaths..."

Branches snagged my sleeves as I crashed through the under-growth. Thin trees loomed overhead and the gray light filtering through made my footing precarious. My breath grew ragged as I struggled to push through. It was just behind me. I couldn't see or hear it, but I knew it was there just the same. Strategy, I thought to myself. There is a way to get out of it. Just think.

Suddenly I was ripped through a shaft of light, blinking into the industrial fluorescent bulbs overhead. Terrified and confused, I bolted upright and tried to pull away whatever vines lingered from the forest and wrapped around my arms. Two strangers rushed over to me, and finally I understood where I was when I saw their scrubs and the tubes attached to my body.

They pushed me back down as I stared at them one by one.

"Shhh. Lie down now, you need some more time to rest." I lay back down and they went back to work. As soon as they turned away, I tried to sit up again, this time getting one leg out of the blanket and preparing to walk out.

My addled brain was thinking, okay this is done. I need to get home now.

They rushed back to push me down again, this time staying close. The man seemed irritated by my misbehavior while the woman was sympathetic and offered, "Are you hungry? Would you like a peanut butter and jelly?"

I thought about the gluten the naturopath I had so eagerly sought the advice of had warned me against and the rash my internist had determined had come from peanut butter.

"No thanks," I muttered. It seemed too much trouble to explain.

"How about some cranberry juice?" the man said, suddenly inter-ested in my well-being again.

Too much sugar, too many additives, probably even red dye. "No, could I have some water?"

"Why don't you want the cranberry juice?"

Surprised by his question, I mulled it over. "Too sweet," I offered, hoping it would satisfy him enough to leave. No such luck.

"Maybe you should stick with the cranberry juice and have a few crackers."

I stared at him, not taking the bait. What was the big deal about water? Requiring that he should move?

"When can I go home?"

"You need a little more time to rest," said the female nurse, who I quickly realized was the nice one, as she looked at my chart. "You've only been out of surgery for an hour. That's pretty fast to wake up. You can take your time."

"No, I think I'm ready. Can you get my husband?"

"Chase will get him," she motioned over to the mean nurse who was typing furiously at his computer station.

He ignored her or was too engrossed in his own thought process to respond.

Instead he countered with, "Can you tell me if you're having any pain?"

I thought it over, my brain reluctantly leaving thoughts of escape and returning to my body. I did a quick scan, then the fog of anesthesia cleared enough to present a sharp pain in the area of my left armpit. "Yes, under my arm hurts."

"On a scale of one to ten, one being very little to ten being the worst pain you ever had, please rate it," he said.

"Um, 8."

"8? 8? It shouldn't be an 8. How would you describe it?" he said doubtfully.

"It really hurts." Lacking any ambition to go into more detail at the searing hot pain that crept under my arm. "Maybe a 7, but I think an 8."

The mean nurse started to argue with me while the nice nurse picked up my chart again. "She's had two babies. I think she knows what an 8 is. Okay, dear, I'm going to get the doctor to give you a little more to manage the pain."

Finally, someone seemed to be speaking my language. "Maybe not too much," I said. I didn't want them to sedate me so much that I had to stay in this alternate reality vortex any longer than absolutely necessary.

"What is your fear?" The mean one asked.

"My fear?" I blinked at him. "I'm not afraid. I just want to get home to my kids."

"Uh huh," he nodded with satisfaction as if my answer had said everything. He then went to his station and struck up a conversation with another young man in scrubs laughing and sitting on the desk, having finally settled his pesky patient.

Just then the surgical intern bounced in gracefully with a big smile. She has way too much energy, I thought with just a slight bit of envy.

"Hi, Aime, how are you feeling?" she asked, grabbing my chart. What did the chart say that everyone was so interested in?

"I'm okay. My left underarm is pretty sore. I wasn't expecting the pain to be so far from my breast."

"Yeah, we had to do a little work with the lymph node area, the tools can reach pretty far from the actual incision, so that will be sore for a while. So the surgery went well. The margins looked pretty good. We tested some nodes and you had three clear ones, but one did test positive. So you'll definitely need to do chemo."

I nodded. "Okay. Thanks." And she bounced away. Chemo. I think I was prepared for that because it didn't seem so much like a shock as a grim acknowledgment.

What seemed like hours later, Scott came rushing in, disheveled from waiting all day.

"Hi," I said, just glad to see him. His face was a mixture of relief, worry, and annoyance.

"Are you doing okay?" he asked, searching my face. I nodded in response. "How long have you been awake?"

"I don't know, an hour?"

"I don't know why it took them so long to come get me. Dr. D came out and talked to me a while ago and I thought they would bring me back then. I've been waiting around this whole time, and I finally found someone to ask to bring me back."

I looked over at the mean nurse, who was rapidly becoming the bad nurse in my mind. He was still chatting with his friend at the desk.

"Do you think we could go? Let's tell them I'm ready" I said, confident that if Scott would agree we could get out of there.

"If you think you're ready," he looked at me with worry lines etched around his eyes.

"I am," I said eagerly, "Just help me look sober."

The good nurse finally agreed after I proved to her that I could go to the bathroom. She gave me some anti-nausea medicine and crackers for the ride home and wished me good luck.

We got home and the kids were still awake. Dad met us at the door, patting my shoulder gently and assuring me that the day had gone well with the kids. I was so relieved to see them both, padding around the house in their socks and pajamas, ready for bed.

They ran to the door, calling, Mama, Mama, and gave me tender hugs. Scott stood beside me in a defensive stance, urging them to be cautious with me. Catherine blanched slightly when she saw me up close, and Wesley plastered a smile, and then ducked into the study to get on the computer.

Well, okay, I thought, back to normal. All the activity had taken my breath away, so I made my way toward the bedroom. Then I looked into the mirror and saw my face the way they had seen it. I was so pale it seemed as if most of the blood had left my body, and the light purple circles I sometimes got under my eyes had turned an ugly brown. I was some ghostly version of myself. I crawled into bed, needing to rest and not even thinking about the food or water I had gone without all day. Then Catherine crawled into bed with me.

"See?" I whispered as I snuggled close to her, brushing her long blonde curls away from her face and touching her cheek. "Everything's fine. It'll just take me a few days to recover." She nodded. Then her eyes turned red and welled up. "What's wrong? I'm fine! Don't worry!"

"I know, it's just that I didn't think it would be like this."

"What do you mean?" I searched her hazel eyes that had turned to a deep olive with the tears.

She paused, then said, "I didn't think it would be so bad."

"I know, honey. But it will be okay."

We cried together curled up under the soft blankets in my bed, my sanctuary. The place where I conceived, labored, and nursed my children. The place of so much love, rest, tears and life. The place that would heal us. During all of our moves, it had been the one constant in our ever-changing lives, our bed.

CHAPTER 8

✤

Nobody Dies From This

I ASK TOO many questions. That's always what has gotten me into trouble. And it's what happened just before Jackie dropped by with her gluten-free baked ziti and salad. She bustled in burdened with bags and an industrial-sized aluminum tin bearing a huge grin that lit up her whole face.

"Hi-ii." She had a habit of drawing out the greeting into two long notes, but by the time she reached the second one, she saw through my own plastered smile that something had happened. Most people couldn't see through my best Southern-bred smile, but Jackie always could.

Her own smile went from genuine to frozen in an instant for the benefit of the kids while she mouthed "What happened?" She tossed everything onto the tile countertop without a second glance and placed her newly unburdened hands on both of my arms, looking up and searching my face for unsaid words.

"Bedroom" she whispered, and we hustled down the hallway before I let it all out in an escalating mode of panic. It was my classic holding it together until someone asked me how I was.

The surgeon had just called about some ultrasound results. He told me how he found the positive node by feel instead of the normal indicators and it seemed to make him nervous, as if it could have been easily missed. He was deliberating between continuing to cut away at lymph nodes and starting chemo right away. He wasn't completely satisfied with either option, and his brutally honest answers to more of my "what if" questions had made me unhappy about the choices too.

Finally, when I got it all out, I stood in front of Jackie, full of fear and questions, "What if it's already spread past the nodes? We know it's on the move because it got that far. It could be anywhere. He said blood, bones... brain..." I stumbled over the last word, an image of my mother's motionless body lying in the hospital room flashing through my head.

"Aime, look at me. We don't know that. We don't know that it's spread. It probably hasn't. There's nothing that has happened yet that's gotten you out of that high success rate. I know you're worried about your mom, but this is totally different. Just do what the doctors say and you'll be fine."

"But they're not sure what's best. What if they made the wrong choice? What if it doesn't work? It's too soon for me! Even Mom got to see all of her children married and so many grandchildren. I can't leave yet! I can't leave the kids. They still need me. Scott will be okay after a while, maybe even Catherine can live on with some scars, but Wesley will not be okay! He is too young, he is too emotional. He still needs me. He will not be okay." Tears started flowing freely as I shook and held onto Jackie.

I gulped some air and wiped my face a little, letting out a nervous laugh, "I'm losing it. Tell me nobody dies from this anymore, right? Nobody!"

Jackie looked back straight into my eyes, still holding both of my arms. "Nobody dies from this." God love her. We both knew she was lying, but she did it convincingly for me.

I pulled myself together and we started back toward the kitchen. She stopped me. "Aime, more importantly *you* will not die from this."

Maybe that last part I could believe.

I spent a couple more days shuffling around the house with my left arm pinned against my side trying to recover, but I still had not hired a baby-sitter to help out with after-school care. I placed an ad on a childcare service I used explaining my circumstances and hoped to find someone who would be comfortable taking care of the kids while I was around. It was a tall order compared to the college kids I usually hired. I needed someone who wouldn't be squeamish about my being sick, who could act normal around the kids, who could drive them around and pick them up from school and help out with light housekeeping.

I got a few responses, but one turned out to be much more than potential childcare. Our email exchange went off like rapid fire:

To: Aime Card
From: Laura Z

Hello There!

My name is Laura and I live in San Carlos.
I may be available to help you but most important, I just wanted you to know in case this is your first time with Chemo? I have been through this too.

I had a lumpectomy, chemo and radiation. How I dealt with cancer was to act like it wasn't a big deal. It was a bump in the road. I was very clear on my intention that…leaving this planet before I am 93 is not an option.
That I believe was the best attitude to have for myself and our 6 kids.
Yes! …..This SUCKS! ….
But it's only a year from our lives where things will be ridiculous around here.
We will get through this and we will all learn great strength and compassion from it.
So that is the Gift you get from cancer.
Also tripping around the house in your jammies for months isn't so bad either.

Everyone processes their fears together as a family.

It's such a teaching time. When they are older they will be the brave friends that are capable of showing up when someone needs them.

Getting the best nutrition into your body and staying hydrated is crucial also.

I never lost my appetite, damn it!! I think I was the first woman to gain mass amounts of weight during chemo! And I still have it. Ugh!

I'll send you some photos.

I cut my hair short, then when it started to fall out I went to the barber shop and shaved it. Nothing felt right to me on my head except a bandana. I didn't want to wear a wig because I think it helps other women know they can go through it and be fine. No need to hide it for others comfort. What about mine? Lol. A bandana felt better than a wig. That's a personal choice everyone makes. It surprised me how significant it felt.

Anyhooooo, lol

If you want I can come by for 30 minutes and we can chat some more if you think I could be helpful.

Talk soon
Sincerely,
Laura

I eagerly kept up the exchange, loving her candid approach and upbeat energy. We ultimately determined the timing didn't work out, but we kept in touch via email.

To: Aime Card
From: Laura Z

Hello Again!

I would love to be your chemo buddy if you like.
The first several treatments are no big deal at all. By my last couple of treatments I insisted on going alone and driving my-self. The nurses are so nice and you are just chilling in your chair like you would be on an airplane but there is an IV in your hand. Bring things to keep you busy or rest or sleep.

The tougher part for me came toward the end when the skin on my tongue got raw.
(But they give you stuff for that) I had several bloody nose in-stances. I broke out with itchy bumps. Basically the build up of the chemo in your system taking its toll on the rest of your body.

I got very cranky feeling. Not toward the family, but my body felt antsy and it made me want to scream. Like I drank 20 cups of coffee and had bad anxiety.
My husband would come home from work and I would just want to crawl in his pocket and cry. Then he would remind me our friends gave me medicinal marijuana. I would take one hit and EVERYTHING was better! I swear By it and recommend it for everyone to have on hand.

Ha ha ha, you were looking for a nanny and you found a drug pusher.

I'm going to send you some photos of me before, bald and after that you can show the kids. Then if I come over to meet them they will see I am back to normal and you will be too.

And PS, all of our kids are grown and five are out of the area. My husband had four and I had two. This was a second marriage for both of us. Like the Brady Bunch. Lol, When I went through cancer in 2010 we had 3 at home. I managed fine.
I will send photos ASAP!
Laura

I pored over Laura's photos and words, hoping and believing that my experience could be like hers. It almost sounded like fun the way she described it. I had thought about the prospect of pot making the whole process easier. I had heard that it could be helpful with nausea for chemotherapy, but I thought it might be even better to help me chill out. There could be advantages to living in California where medical marijuana was legal, after all. I started doing some research, and after seeing the results of studies that had shown a significant decrease in tumor size in mice, I was willing to give it a try.

That Saturday morning Scott and I drove to a medical marijuana clinic right in downtown San Carlos, and after a quick meeting with the doctor, I officially had my pot card. I still keep it in my wallet for fun.

CHAPTER 9

I Have a Plan

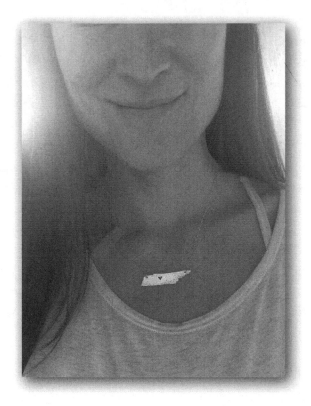

I ASKED JACKIE, Lauren and Shelley over to my house on Saturday. Scott and Dad needed to get the kids out of the house as they were all getting a little stir crazy, and I knew it would do everyone some good to have a change of scene for the afternoon. They both cleaned up as well as they could, which for them is basically throwing the dishes in the dishwasher and putting things in strategically placed piles to be dealt with (by me) at some point in the future. They all eagerly agreed to head to Pescadero to see the ocean and play around in the sand. After a whirl-wind of activity and rounding up Maverick, they were off. The house was strangely silent without them, but the silence came as a relief.

There had been an unusual number of texts and emails tossed around among the girls regarding a pajama party. Shelley, ever the fashionista, didn't seem to get it.

Shelley: So you wear your pajamas during the day?
Jackie: Yes.
Shelley: You mean I walk out of my house wearing pajamas.
Aime: Yes.
Shelley: Are we talking robe and slippers or just pj's?
Jackie: Whatever you want.
Shelley: Could I bring my pajamas and put them on there?
Aime: That's fine.
Shelley: The things I am willing to do for Aime ....
Shelley: What should I bring?
Jackie: We are thinking quiches, champagne etc.
Shelley: You want me to cook a quiche? How do I do that?
Jackie: It's easy.
Shelley: Easy for you to say it's easy. So what should I bring?
Aime: How about a fruit salad?
Shelley: I can do that.

I bustled around myself, changing from my yoga pants to some paja-mas with little heart faces and cheeky moustaches all over them that I had bought in anticipation of my surgery. Then I headed back up to the kitchen to straighten up. The plan was for the girls to bring the food, so I just needed to have things cleared and set up for a lunch. I laughed to myself at Dad wrinkling his nose at my idea of a pajama party in the afternoon.

"They don't know you've been getting dressed every day for a week already," he huffed a little, bristling at my enthusiasm to embrace my invalid state. Okay, Dad, I thought, if you call throwing on my yoga pants getting dressed, then I will too.

Knocking at the door interrupted my thoughts, and I hurried over to let Lauren in, bearing gluten-free quiches from Zest, a bakery I had recently discovered in San Carlos that made gluten-free everything.

"Wow, thank you!" I nodded toward the signature pink bakery boxes. "What a yummy treat!"

"I know, I love them," Lauren said as she put them on the counter and plopped onto a stool. She had let her long red hair stay in its naturally curly state and she scraped it back off her face into a pony tail. "I got two meat and two veggie, so we can either split them up or decide who wants what."

"I'm fine with either, so we'll just see what everyone wants to do." I shrugged, turning on the oven to heat them up. "I made some fruit tea this morning. I figured this would be a perfect time for it. Our very civilized pajama luncheon."

"Oh, warning," Lauren said. "Shelley was very confused as to the type of fruit that should go in the salad, so I spent a lot of time with her on the phone this morning coaching her through the Trader Joe's experience. I don't think she had ever been in one before. I told her the fruit had to be organic and that really freaked her out."

I laughed at the thought of Shelley fumbling through Trader Joe's searching for organic strawberries in her heels. "Oh, that's so mean! We should have given her something easier."

"Something easier than cut fruit? You can buy it that way."

Another knock at the door announced the arrival of Jackie and Shelley, who let themselves in and called, "Hello!" as they made their way back to the kitchen. Jackie burst into the room with her best smile, fully decked out in a leopard print pajama set the exact color of her honey brown hair. She had a bowl of salad greens under her arm and waved a bottle of good champagne at me.

"I had a feeling this day might call for something stronger than tea," she winked.

"Absolutely!" I happily agreed. "Toss it in the fridge and that will be our dessert!"

Shelley came in behind her and I gave her a big hug. She tugged at her pajamas nervously, "This is the first time I have ever been out of the house in my pajamas *in my life,* and I want you to know that I am doing this for you."

I giggled at her and held out my hand for the package of strawberries she was grasping. "And I greatly appreciate the effort it took you. I think, however, that the fancy monogramming makes up for some of the informality." I said, taking in the silk pajamas with contrasting piping and velvet slides.

"Oh, that's okay. Let me wash them." Shelley rushed over to the sink and gave the strawberries a thorough rinsing. I handed her a strainer and she stuffed the packaging way down in the recycle bin as if she were worried she hadn't gotten the right kind.

"Okay, so I wasn't able to cook a quiche, but I can do some things," Shelley pronounced proudly as she looked at her beautifully washed and ripened strawberries. "You know, just this week I made powdered donuts for E's school."

"Really?" Jackie piped in. "That's impressive!"

"Yes I did. I took regular donuts and shook them in a baggy with powdered sugar and presto! Powdered donuts!"

Lauren snorted behind her hand and Jackie burst out laughing.

"Oh, it's so fun to have you all here! What a perfect way to spend our Saturday!" I said as I looked at their smiling faces filling up my kitchen.

"Are you kidding me? It's my pleasure! And as an added bonus, I got out of James's baseball double header today." Jackie laughed. "Where should we set up?"

"Let's eat out on the deck," I gestured toward the open door. "It's such a beautiful day."

We had a healthy lunch of quiche, green salad, and strawberries, then we moved to the cushioned chairs, still wanting to enjoy the sun and the bright blue sky.

"Do you find out about schools for Catherine this week?" Lauren asked as she sat down in one of the lounge chairs.

"Friday," I said. "I'm trying not to worry about it, everyone assured me it should be fine so I'm going to believe them. It's a little nerve-wracking because she just applied to two schools, but she's such a good student." I trailed off and looked out over the trees.

Jackie jumped in, "Stop. It's going to be fine. She's absolutely precious, all the schools should be dying to have her."

A cloud seemed to pass over our day with the mention of the stressful topic. It was the dirty little secret of competitiveness that was common to most of the private schools in Silicon Valley- the ability to help the children move on to the next rung of the ladder toward a great college. Our strategy of applying to only two schools had made a little more sense when we lived in Woodside with a sweet and small public elementary school as a backup, but the San Carlos middle school was a really big place that might be harder for a new student to assimilate to.

"So, Lauren, what do you think of this crazy place? Have you met anyone that works at Google yet?" Jackie asked, clearly eager to change the conversation.

"No, why?" Lauren asked.

"It's a short conversation, but humorous. They won't tell you anything about what they do. It's like they work for the CIA," Jackie said with a snicker.

"Oh, I know," I said. "They're the first to tell you where they work because they're so proud of it, but then they refuse to answer any questions. It's weird."

"This whole place is weird but intoxicating," Lauren said. "There is so much happening here. When people tell you that they're having a big week, you'll hear about it on the news. Not the local news, the national news. But I'm having trouble putting my finger on the culture. I mean the social expectations."

"Hah," Jackie said. "That's because there aren't any."

"I felt the same way," I said to Lauren. "I was looking for this code of conduct to figure out how to fit in, but it doesn't exist. It's such a recent blend of so many different cultures that no one way to behave has prevailed."

I'd felt the pressure to keep up with the Jones' everywhere I'd lived, but it was never more present than in Silicon Valley. In the South, it was also important to be considered a "good family," which was why the question "Where do you go to church?" was socially acceptable. In New England one also gained status from being "an old family." Descendants from an old family might never do anything notable again but inherit the benefit of social status. In Silicon Valley, neither of those things were important at all. The things that mattered were a person's resume and the cash they earned—proven by cars, homes, vacations, and the success of their children, the ultimate goal being getting them through Stanford to run startups of their own. Each step of the ladder—private schools, special programs, accolades—that the children reached demonstrated one's success toward that end goal. I had fallen into it. I wanted to fit in, and I wanted all of us to succeed.

"So what happened with the whole benefit thing?" Jackie asked when the conversation paused.

Lauren and Shelley filled her in, each cautious of their words, careful not to offend each other and maybe a little embarrassed to tell Jackie exactly how it had played out.

"What a nightmare!" Jackie said and rolled her eyes. "And that is exactly why I don't work on the benefit. I got burned with the raffle the first year and then I chalked it up as a waste of time."

"I know," I said. "It seems so much more efficient to just write a check and save everyone all the time and hassle. But it is nice to have some kind of community event—a reason for the parents to go out without the kids and socialize."

"And to wear a pretty dress, of course," Shelley piped in. "I always love a reason to wear a pretty dress. Speaking of, what are you wearing this year?" she asked me.

"I really don't think I'll be able to go." I said, even though by then I had told her a couple of times already. "It just depends on my schedule and the timing of everything." I deliberately left *everything* vague, not wanting the thought of chemo to spoil my afternoon.

"Well, I'm going to save a spot for you anyway. Just in case," she said, nodding her head at me and raising her eyebrows as if to influence my decision.

Jackie seemed to keep a close eye on my energy, checking in on me to make sure I wasn't getting tired. I wasn't. In fact, it was wonderfully energizing to have some real girl time for the afternoon. We finished the tea and brought out the champagne and toasted to our health.

The next Tuesday I had my follow-up appointment with Dr. D to make sure everything was healing up well from the surgery and my initial meeting with the oncologist. Once you're in the system at the Stanford Cancer Center, the doctors like to keep you with their team. The office spaces are all together in the same section of the building, and the nurses told me that they often confer on patient strategy while just meeting each other in the hallways. Another patient I met in the waiting area had assured me that I was in the right place. "Start talking to other patients and you'll see. They come here from all over. More often than not, they've started treatment somewhere else, and when a complication happens, they end up here. If you have the opportunity to start out here, it's a no-brainer."

An added patient benefit was that I could go to one place and even stay in the same exam room while meeting with both the surgeon and the oncologist. So that was how it happened that Scott and I spent the day finding out how the next several months might play out for us. The info drip had begun.

The surgeon went over the path report in detail. The tumor was actually a little smaller than they thought, which would have reduced my stage from two to one, but one lymph node was full of cancer cells and there were isolated cells in another, which bumped my stage back up to two. Another factor was that the tumor was placed just a hair too close to the skin for him to take the margin of tissue away that is ideal, so I would need to have a follow-up surgery after chemotherapy.

He shrugged a little sheepishly and said, "I know it's not ideal to have to have another surgery, but I think it's worth it to make sure nothing is left behind." He seemed to be happy to have the excuse to get back in and have another go at those troublesome lymph nodes. "I can also go back in with the same incision site, so you won't be left with another scar." Somehow it reassured me that he was thinking ahead about aesthetics because the last on my list of worries was the presence of an extra scar on my breast. The only reason I was relieved to be able to keep my breasts at all was because the more invasive surgery had a longer recovery time. Otherwise I would have been ready to just let them go.

At that point, all I wanted to hear was that I would live. When I pushed him for a definitive, Dr. D countered with a straightforward and honest philosophy that I embraced. "There is always a certain amount of risk. Life itself carries no guarantees. I could walk out the door and get hit by a car today. We just do what we can to minimize our risk, and then the rest is left to fate. Or faith."

The surgical team left saying that we would meet again toward the end of chemo to discuss the next surgery. At the time it just felt like a date on the calendar, but what I didn't realize was that between those two meetings my body would be taken to the very edge of life, and I would be forced to stare out at the chasm. Some parting words from the surgeon stuck with me:

"Right now we don't know for sure how well the chemo will work for each particular patient, but what we do know is that in total it gives each person the best odds, so we do it. Right now it's the best we have."

Scott and I then passed an anxious half an hour or so while we waited on Dr. S, the oncologist I had yet to meet. I sat on the cold table crinkling up the paper lining as I shifted around restlessly in my gown, and Scott sat in one of the chairs beside the exam table compulsively checking his phone. He didn't talk about it, but I knew it worried him to see the work piling up while he took these hours and days with me. He wasn't a salaried employee; he was a mergers and acquisitions advisor who worked solely on commission. He brought in the deals himself and worked them all the way through to the end. He only got paid if the deals closed, and since he worked mostly on the sell side, only if his clients—the companies he worked with—ultimately sold. It was a feast or famine job, and it took a disciplined approach to savings and a steel gut to survive. Now he layered in worries about my health along with constant financial concerns, and I could see the strain in the darkening circles that were growing under his eyes.

Finally there was a knock on the exam door and Dr. S came in, reaching out her hand in greeting.

"Okay, so here we are. I'm sorry that you have to be here, but we're going to do everything it takes to get you back to your life." She looked to be about my age and like any one of the other moms I might know from school. She had her curly dark hair pulled back and she wore street clothes. The only giveaway that announced she was a doctor was the stethoscope thrown casually around her neck. "So let's talk. Based on the pathology from your surgery and taking into consideration your young age and vitality, it's clear that we should recommend to you what we consider the gold standard of chemotherapy. This is four rounds taking place over the course of eight weeks of a combination of Adriamycin and Cytoxan followed by twelve weekly doses of Taxol for a total of twenty weeks of chemotherapy. After three to four weeks of recovery, you'll have your follow-up surgery, and after that the standard is five weeks of radiation."

Scott was writing notes, rapidly trying to keep up, and we immediately started counting the weeks on the calendar. After a few questions we determined that if everything went as expected, we could be wrapping this up by Halloween, Thanksgiving at the latest.

"Okay," I responded, somehow energized by being able to see an end date. "So this is doable. How much of this is total down time versus what I might be able to power through?"

"It's hard to say until we find out how your body responds," Dr. S responded. "Each person is different. However, I can say that typically the most difficult part is the Adriamycin and Cytoxan, which we call AC, which will be the first eight weeks. With that you can expect some more severe symptoms such as nausea, loss of appetite, and fatigue, but it's not for the entire time. Typically patients start feeling better in time for the next round. That's the idea anyway. And that's part of what makes it difficult. Just when you're starting to feel normal again, it starts all over. The last twelve rounds of Taxol tend to be tolerated much more easily, so for those last few weeks you should start to feel better, but with weekly dosing it's more of a constant level of symptoms until the cumulative effect starts to build up in the end. The good news is that you should start to see some hair regrowth during Taxol."

"Oh, so I will lose my hair? Dr. D had suggested that I might be able to use the ice caps. I did a little research on the possibility, and to me they seemed doable." We were treading on delicate territory as we spoke about my hair. I had been holding onto the ice cap idea, thinking that with my thick hair, I could lose half, and it would still look relatively normal.

"Yes. Hair loss is one of the unfortunate side effects. Many people think it is the worst one. You can try the ice caps if you like. I have seen people do it, and they can help you with that at the infusion center." She looked at my hairline and kept her expression carefully guarded. "But I would suggest that it is a lot of pain and hassle and with this particular treatment often doesn't work very well. You would have to have someone trained to handle the rotation of the caps during and after each round of chemotherapy, and with this regimen and for you it is unlikely that you will get much of a result."

Just the day before I had told another mom at school about the ice cap idea, and she had said, "Oh good. You have to keep your hair. You have great hair. So do I, so I can say that. When you have great hair you have to keep it. It's part of who you are."

I had responded, "Oh, thanks. I know. It's like it's part of my identity." Even as I said the words I felt a butterfly flip in my stomach. It was superstition, but it felt like I was tempting fate to say the words out loud. Part of my identity. I understood the superstition better after going to my first Red Sox game with Scott. When I cheerfully talked about their winning the game before it was over, he winced at me while the guys behind us scowled and grumbled.

Scott explained to me that you can't talk about being ahead during the game or you might jinx the team. I laughed at the idea that I would have anything to do with the outcome of the game, but just then the opposing team hit a home run, tying the game, and the Sox ended up losing in the ninth inning by one. Walking out of Fenway Park, the crowd was quiet from the disappointing finish and I heard a salty old New Englander say to his son in his thick Boston accent, "That's the Red Sox for ya. They'll break your heart every time." Of course that was before the curse was broken.

"Okay," I looked at Scott, knowing the ice cap idea would be too much to expect of him for only a chance of keeping part of my hair, and I reluctantly gave up on the whole idea. "So I lose my hair during the AC, and it starts to come back during Taxol, so really it'll just be a couple of months wearing wigs or something. I guess I can do that."

Dr. S gave a noncommittal shrug, knowing I would be without my hair for far more time than my estimation. "The important thing to keep in mind is that all of this is leading you toward the goal of saying you are cured. I think that is a powerful word, cured, and we are not afraid to use it. It is possible, even likely, for you to be cured by the end of the year."

I know it sounds crazy, but for the first time in the whole process I felt with some certainty that I would actually survive, and it was such a relief.

"Okay," I said. "I can do this. A few months of feeling sick and then it's all behind us. Let's do it." I smiled at Scott and he smiled back and nodded, catching my enthusiasm.

They saw the optimistic looks passing between us and Dr. S spoke up, asking if we'd given any thoughts to our plans, our strategy. "So do you have enough support at home?"

Scott and I looked at each other, and I shrugged. "We're lining up some help now. I think we'll be okay."

"That's good. Just remember, there are a lot of resources you can take advantage of through Stanford and in the community in general. I know this can put a particularly difficult strain on young families. Just know that you can reach out to us if you ever feel like you need it." She looked back and forth between the two of us.

"Thanks," Scott said and nodded.

We wrapped up the details and said our goodbyes. Dr. S later told me that when she left the room she let out a nervous laugh and told her RN, "She scares me." When her nurse asked her why, she admitted the truth of it, "Because we're going to bring her so low. It's such a long way to fall."

On the way home Scott and I decided the way that it would be... mapping out the chemo days, being cautious with his time away from work, and outsourcing as much as possible. I thought we could manage.

> From: Aime Card
> Date: Tuesday, March 11, 2014
> Subject: I have a Plan!
>
> Hello ladies,
>
> I just wanted to give you an update because I'm so relieved I finally have a plan! The bad news is I'm going to have to do the heavy duty chemo. But the good news is that all my doctors feel good about our plan and are taking this approach as a 40 year clear plan. In other words because of my age and this particular cancer's aggressive nature they have to go all in, but the aggressiveness of it makes it very highly treatable. Sort of ironic. So they're going in all guns blazing and they'll catch any potential stray cells now and keep it from recurring.
>
> Long and short—chemo starts in 2–3 weeks. I'll be sick for the better part of 8 weeks—then for the next 12 I'll be slightly less sick. So 20 weeks of chemo, then one more minor surgery, 5 weeks of radiation and I'll be free and clear! So we will have a very merry Christmas.
>
> Love to you all!!!
> xoxox
> Aime

I sent out the email to my group of close friends here and back East that I wanted to keep in the loop. I was surprised by the range of responses. Shock, prayer, sending love. But, No! I wanted to respond back. Don't you see? It's going to be okay! Yes, I have a lot in front of me, but it's going to be fine! Scott and I had talked it out. We had a plan. It was all going to be just fine.

Then the next day reality started to sink in. I had been so relieved to have a plan and to finally believe that I might live through it. Then I was faced with the realization that these next few months were really going to suck.

Jackie called me and said, "Okay, girl. We're going to get you through this. Give me the list. Tell me what you need."

A few hours later I sat back and looked at the Word document I had put together trying to get myself and my thoughts organized. It was filled with a succession of household tasks and kids activities, and red lined with days that I anticipated being unavailable. Maverick to daycare, Catherine to riding, bone scans, CT scans, port placement, Wesley's lacrosse practice, chemo. Outsourcing cleaning and laundry. Kids, dog, chemo.

Okay, I thought to myself. It looks like a lot, but I can do this. This is a finite number of tasks. We will get through it. Somehow.

I wondered how it even got set up that way. I had to think about it to reinforce my original decisions about what activities were right for each kid and how much we did that was optional. I decided to keep the kids' activities going. They were going to need to stay busy and keep as much of their lives as constant as they could.

Looking at my life on paper, I was astonished by what even the bare minimum consisted of. Was that the sum total of my life? Was that what I was living for, what I wanted to live for? Driving the kids around and keeping up with someone else's expectations of what it meant to be a good mother, a good wife, a good person?

I closed my laptop shutting off the white glare of the page.

CHAPTER 10

Middle School Fiasco

I CLEANED UP what was left in the sink the best I could with one arm held gingerly against my chest, still sore from the surgery. I leaned down to flip the dishwasher door up and caught sight of Dad lounging out on the deck, finishing off his sandwich. That's right, I thought. It's a beautiful day, he's leaving tomorrow, and we just have an hour before we need to pick up the kids, so I walked out and plopped down in my favorite cushioned deck chair beside him. The sun filtered through the trees dotting our heads with just the right amount of light to keep the temperature comfortable.

It had been such an enormous help to have him with me these past couple of weeks. It was more than I had ever hoped he could provide. He had spent the past year just trying to get his feet under him after the months of caring for Mom and then finally coping with being alone for the first time in his life. He had to learn everything from how to cook to how to do laundry. I had seen Fronda's carefully written instructions for laundry taped up on the wall next to the washing machine the last time I had been in his house, and he had called me once from a Trader Joe's, where he sounded a little lost while he searched for the particular kind of bread he liked. When he came to California to help me, I was expecting him to just drive the kids around and maybe supervise the dinners, but he jumped in like a champ. The previous night I had seen him on his knees in front of the washer and dryer folding my laundry. I had never seen him do that before, and it struck me as beautiful and melancholy at the same time. That was never the role I wanted him to fill. I wanted my mom for that.

I turned my face up to the sun and sighed.

"Nice day," Dad said between bites of chips. "You know, I really love this view." He gestured out over the canyon. "What did you say this area is called again?"

Everyone always commented on the nice days when they came to visit from back East. We had already come to take them for granted, accepting in stride the easy climate that Scott referred to as a "weather vacuum" when we first moved. "It's like there's no weather at all. It feels the same inside and out. It's like a total absence of weather," he, being a hard core New Englander, had lamented one day when he was still adjusting to the move.

"Devonshire Canyon. I know, this is really my favorite part of the house. I spend a lot of time out here," I smiled back at Dad and leaned back into my chair, looking up at the eucalyptus leaves that hung overhead. We spent a few moments in companionable silence while he ate, gazing over the water oak tree tops that grazed the railing of the deck and out toward the ridgeline dotted with homes.

My phone interrupted the silence, and I glanced down to see a number I didn't recognize. "I'd better get this," I said, thinking it could be a doctor or anyone, really. I didn't have the luxury of screening calls anymore.

"Hello?"

"Oh, Aime. I wasn't sure if I would catch you. It's Rachael from Episcopal School."

"Oh hi, Rachael. How are you?" My heart skipped a beat. Getting calls from the kids' school during the day is always a bit unsettling.

"The kids are fine," she assured me. "I always have to start a conversation that way," she said. "It's just how parents worry."

"Oh good. So what's going on?" I asked.

"Well, it's about Catherine. I just heard from the schools about their admissions lists, and I didn't want you to have to wait for the mail tomorrow to hear the news. It turns out that she was wait-listed to both schools she applied to."

"Oh no," my heart sank, brain reeling, going into bad-news-received/information-gathering mode. This was getting to be an all too familiar response.

"I wanted to let you know so you could think how best to prepare Catherine for the news. She will be in the position where friends of hers will have been accepted, so we feel that it is best in these cases for her to be told the news instead of having to open up the letter."

The mental image of Catherine waiting for the mail delivery and then excitedly opening up the envelopes only to get her hopes dashed crushed me.

"Yes, I agree with you there. So, what do you think our plan should be now? Do you think she is likely to come off the wait list? How long does this process last, and should we simultaneously start looking at other options?"

"Well, both schools told me that she is highly qualified, which we already knew, and that on her own she is placed high on each wait list. The accepted applicants have one week to decide, and then there should be movement on the wait lists. I hope I am not steering you wrong here, but I feel very confident that she will get into one if not both of the schools off of the wait list. Quite frankly, I am very surprised that she didn't get accepted."

"Do you have a sense of what happened?" I asked, still absorbing the shock and sense of hurt on Catherine's behalf.

"The only thing I heard was that at Holy Cross she was quiet during her shadow day and they had a difficult time judging her interest level."

"Oh, no. That is such a shame, because Holy Cross was actually the school that she preferred. I remember telling you during our conference in the fall that I was most concerned about the shadow because of how reserved she is in new situations. It's tough to expect a fifth grader to be able to overcome personality traits for an interview process like this." I stopped myself from saying it, but I also remembered that when I had voiced my concern in our fall conference Rachael had nodded confidently, responding, "Well, that's where we come in and can tell the schools what we know about the children."

"Oh, I know. It's really too much to expect from an eleven-year-old. It's just become such a crazy process. I have known the admissions director at Holy Cross for a long time now, and I might have stepped out of line a bit, but I told him that he made a mistake about this one. And I hope you don't mind, but I told him about your situation as well. He said I was breaking his heart."

"Yes, it is a lot for our family to handle right now. Okay, I apologize if I am being too direct, but the situation I am looking at is that I have two weeks until I have to start chemotherapy, and tomorrow I have a minor surgery to have my port placed and will be out of reach for a few hours. So I need to know exactly what I can do between now and then. We are not considering the public school in San Carlos an option. Catherine doesn't know anyone here yet, and the middle school here is huge. With her being so reserved in new situations, we really feel that it's not the right environment for her. So what do we need to do? Should we ask people to speak for Catherine? Should we start looking at other schools? Which ones do you think would even be options for late applications?"

"Aime, I feel confident that we can take care of this. Let's wait this out one week, and if there is no movement from the wait lists, then we will start looking into other options."

We wrapped up the call, and I leaned back into the chair.

"Everything okay?" Dad asked.

I looked out over the canyon, breathed in the eucalyptus and bay leaves, and let out a long sigh as I leaned my head back against the cushions.

"I guess not. Catherine has been wait-listed to both of the schools she applied to. That was the head of school calling to let me know."

"Oh, no, really?" His dark brows pinched up as if in pain, a familiar sympathetic expression I had seen hundreds of times in my life, which never failed to soothe me. "Did she recommend anything you need to do about it?"

"She said I could call any friends at the schools, but I only know a couple of families at each school. She thinks it's going to be okay." I sighed again, pained at the thought of the extra strain on all of us. "It's just one more thing to add to the task list, and one more thing to worry about, I guess."

"I'm sorry, sweetie." His kind hazel eyes locked into mine, and he leaned over and patted my knee.

I called Scott and let him know. I could tell his frustration was running pretty close to the surface from the tension in his voice. We worked together a quick plan to tell Catherine the next afternoon when I got back from the port placement and her other friends would be finding out. Rachael had told me that some of her friends had been accepted to both schools, but she didn't share the details about which friends or which schools. We also tried to figure out who we might call that could put in a good word for us. I knew the families at the other schools better than he did, so we agreed that I should send emails as opposed to calling, so he could be kept in the loop. He swore softly under his breath, and before I hung up, I think I heard him throw something in his office.

Dad dropped me off at the hospital the next morning before he left for the airport. "Are you sure you don't want me to go in with you?" he asked when he pulled the car up to the door.

"That's okay. You need to go catch your flight. It's been so great to have you here, Dad. Thanks so much for coming. It made such a difference for the kids, so they could have some fun Papa time instead of just worrying about me."

"I'm just glad I could help out. And you know I always love hanging out with the kids. They're really great kids." He smiled and leaned over to give me a hug. "Good luck today. Let me know how it goes."

"Okay, thanks. Have a safe flight." I kissed his cheek and hopped out of the car. The automatic doors whooshed out of the way when I walked through, the vents blew my hair, and I wiped my tears away before anyone could see.

Off he went and I was alone again. My independent nature wasn't working out so well for me anymore.

I was thrown off balance by how similar the check-in process for this "minor procedure" was to my surgery. I was taken to the same prep area, and the staff came around to discuss what would happen. When the oncologist had recommended the port, it seemed like just a little thing to do that would make the chemo infusions easier on my veins, so I agreed, taking their word for it.

The anesthesiologist assured me that I would remain awake throughout the process and that the whole thing should only take a few minutes once we got started. I was wheeled into a surgical room, and he was right, it was very fast. The nurse saw my phone with headphones on my lap and asked if I wanted her to play my music through the sound system. I readily agreed, but I think my playlist only cycled through a few songs before the whole thing was over and I was being wheeled back to recovery.

The surgeon handed me a mirror so I could see where he had placed the port. He seemed proud of his work. I felt the lump mid-way between my right breast and clavicle. It was covered with surgical tape and slightly swollen. I cautiously pressed my fingers into my skin and felt the edges of the device that was shaped like a grape sliced in half with the round side protruding from my chest. I felt a dull pain around the base of my neck as if I had slept on a rock. Upon closer inspection

I saw a smaller piece of tape covering a tiny incision in that area just above my clavicle bone.

"Oh," I said, sickened. He had fished the tube connected to the base of the port under the skin all the way up to and into my jugular vein like an electrician wiring cables through old walls.

The pain started throbbing. "It hurts more than I thought it would," I said.

"Does it? Well, in 20 percent of cases it can cause some discomfort at first. You'll want to take a Vicodin if it hurts already," he said. "Do you have enough? I can write you another prescription for backup."

I called Scott to let him know that I was finished early while the nurse assured me I should wait in recovery for some time for the anesthesia to wear off. Scott was tense, though he tried not to let it show. We hadn't known that the process would be so involved. No one had really explained it. He was frustrated at being caught off guard. We started to realize they would tell us only the barest essential information. I'm not sure exactly what the theory behind the info drip strategy was, but I imagine that if anyone was given the full story from the beginning they would run for the hills. I would have. Then again, sometimes it's better to have more information to be prepared. The bottom line was that either way it was going to suck. Really bad. And for a very long time.

Scott texted me when he drove onto Stanford's campus to let me know he was close, so the nurse walked down with me to meet him and the whole thing was done. I was still numb from the anesthesia and felt fine besides the dull ache in my neck, so we agreed to pick up the kids from school on the way home. Shelley had been on call to bring them home if needed, but I knew that Catherine was anxious to get home and find out about middle schools, so we had that conversation to look forward to. I was using all of my energy to clear my head so I could be available for her.

Catherine jumped into the car, full of excitement. All of the kids had been talking about school news all day. They had been coached to expect some of them to be in wait-list situations and that it would take a little time before some of the children wanted to share their news.

"We are getting notifications from schools in the mail today," she said. "What time do you think it will be there?"

I looked at Scott, and he nodded. Let's just go ahead and burst the bubble, he seemed to say. Her excitement was excruciating to both of us.

"Well, Mrs. Hanlon called me to let me know what happened so that you wouldn't have to wait for your letter. Do you want me to tell you?" I turned around to see her better.

"She did? Okay." She smoothed back her hair and her expression became guarded.

"It turns out that you have been put on the wait list for both schools, which I guess is good news and bad. The good news is that both of the schools think you would be a great addition to their sixth grade classes, but they had so many that they needed to accept, that we will need to wait a little while longer to see if they have space."

"Both of them said that?"

"They did. Remember that the schools have to give priority to kids that have siblings at the school and whose parents work there or went there when they were kids. And there are a lot of people in the area who have personal connections that we don't have yet because we are new here. But the main thing to remember is that both of the schools think you are more than qualified to attend. It's just a matter of space."

I started questioning all of my decisions, like my misguided confidence that because Catherine was a smart, sweet girl with a great work ethic she would be able to get into a decent middle school. I wondered if I had changed my Boston phone number to a local one, or at least had a landline, it would have made us seem like we were more committed to staying. The fact was that I had significantly underestimated the psychotic level of competitiveness that was pervasive in the Silicon Valley private school system.

What I should have done was play the game, hint at big donations, call in favors from anyone I knew. I guessed that was what it took, but in reality I didn't have anything more to bring to the table. We weren't especially well connected, we didn't have a well-funded charitable foundation capable of underwriting new programs for the school, and when I stepped back a moment, I wondered if it really made sense anyway. Do I really want my kids spending time in this environment? A pay-to-play system where the general expectations were nothing short of perfection? When what we as fully functioning adults should convey to our children is that perfection is unattainable for humans?

There was nothing wrong with aiming high, but something was out of whack there. Even the dentist had suggested that Catherine have surgery on her gums to remove a little piece of skin that was creating a very slight gap between her front teeth. We talked about it and agreed that the gap was so minor it wasn't worth the surgery to fix it. Catherine had told me that she liked the gap, and I agreed. It was something that made her unique, like the little freckle on her cheek. This quest for perfection that was pervasive in the culture was more than a little off-putting. But there I was, falling onto the treadmill, being a part of the frantic rat race, and I hated it. I hated what it was doing to the kids and to us. But I couldn't see another way.

Scott glanced back at her in the rearview mirror, and then looked at me. His expression tightened, but he remained quiet, judging Catherine's reaction.

She sat quietly for a moment, and then asked, "How does the wait list work?"

"Some kids will be accepted into more than one school they applied to. They have one week to decide which school they want to attend, and then they will free up a spot at the school they don't choose. So we should start to hear things within the next couple of weeks."

"Okay," she said and remained quiet for several minutes.

"Google car!" Wesley shouted, his voice cutting through the palpable tension in the air.

We all stayed silent.

"Look, look!" He jabbed at the window with his finger pointing out the car beside us with the gigantic antenna on its roof.

"Shhhh,"I started to quiet him then Catherine burst in, "Shut up, Wesley!"

"Hey," Scott said in a gentle rebuke.

I stared at the car going by, this one a Lexus SUV labeled boldly with Google Self-Driving signs. What is this place? This place where we are surrounded by the technology of the future and yet an eleven-year-old straight-A student can get boxed out of private school for being too quiet and because her parents can't afford to give a five hundred thousand-dollar donation? That was the number I had heard casually mentioned over a glass of wine once. That a donation of five hundred thousand could assure a spot at certain schools.

We got home and the kids split off to have snacks and some down time. I caught back up with Catherine later in her room.

"You okay, love?" I sat down on her bed, smoothing out the cheerful turquoise polka-dotted bedspread.

"Yeah, I'm fine." She nodded, looking up from her homework. "It's just frustrating to have to wait longer."

"I know." I put my arm around her shoulders and pulled her into a hug. She stayed close for a moment before pushing away.

"I texted Kiki and she said she got into Holy Cross but not Menlo or Casti."

"Oh, so she'll be at Holy Cross?"

"Yeah. That'll be fun if we can go together. I haven't heard from anyone else yet."

"Okay, well, just try not to worry about it too much. We're going to work really hard to find the right place for you next year. Maybe there are even some other options that we haven't thought of yet. It will all work out."

"I just want to be sure that I go somewhere that I have a friend."

"I know, sweetheart. We'll figure something out. Don't worry," I kissed her head and got up. My neck was throbbing where the port was placed. "I'm going to go rest now. Just come and get me if you want to talk some more, okay?"

"Okay," she said and gave me a brave smile that quivered a little around the edges.

My heart tore as I climbed into bed and pulled the covers over my head. I had less than two weeks until I started chemo.

6:00 p.m.

Shelley: Hi Aime – Just checking in to see how you are feeling. Xo

Aime: Thanks. Was feeling great earlier, but now I want to unleash a tirade of obscenities that I'm sure you don't want to hear. This was supposed to be an easy part. I have this lump under my skin on my chest bone—it's sore and it's f---ing weird!

Shelley: Would any pain meds help? You can call me and yell obscenities. I did that earlier about a client. ☺

Aime: ;) I think my mini rant helped. I took a pain killer at 4. Need to wait a little longer. I think my mistake was telling the anesthesia guy to keep it light because I wanted to be clear this afternoon. I'm going to make a policy of not turning down drugs in the future. Where is my pot delivery guy?

Shelley: Yes, where is that pot delivery guy? Jerk off better get on schedule or he will have to answer to Team Aime and Hubby's!

Aime: I just had to look up the side effects of mixing pot with pain killers. Man, that took me to a weird chat room.
Shelley: Hahahahaha. Please share
Aime: It was all—dude I took two percocets and then my cousin brought some heavy buds and I went blind for 15 seconds.
Shelley: Hahaha. I would be so happy with two percocets.
Aime: I haven't gotten out of bed. Scott is wandering around upstairs I have no idea what he's doing?
Shelley: Is he looking for a beer, maybe?
Aime: I don't know—I hope he's feeding himself and the kids.
Aime: My dad left today ☹
Shelley: Sorry. ☹

9:00 p.m.
Shelley: Hope some meds kicked in. If not, take some more. Sleep well. We are around working/running errands this weekend. Let us know if there is anything we can take off your to do list so you guys can hang out together or relax, okay?

On Sunday I woke up to a text from Lauren.

Lauren: Hiya! Hope ur having a great weekend. Wanted to get the MCC riding summer camp info from you if you have it.
Aime: will send it. Feel like crap from the port placement on Friday ☹
Lauren: Oh no, where is it?
Aime: Right on my bony collar bone. I think that and my tense neck is the issue. If they'd put it in my fat ass I'd have been fine :P
Lauren: hahahaha!! Well not so sure about that though…. You up for a fun outing this week?
Aime: not sure. Schedule is getting tight and I need to bank my rest. What were you thinking?

Lauren: museum and lunch might be low key and nice? Or could do hair apt if you still want to do that. Also up for going to movie if there are any out you want to see.

Aime: I'm going to wait for hair – going to crop it right before chemo on the 25th. What do you think of the robin wright style on house of cards for me? Season 1.

Lauren: love her hair. I think you've got the face to pull it off. You have got to be attractive and you've got that covered!

Aime: It's only going to last a couple of weeks anyway. Smile

Lauren: Also could do Fioli and lunch.

Aime: what's fioli?

Lauren: It's the house and gardens by you. It's gorgeous this time of year and so peaceful. They have a great café too. Or I could just come by and visit if that works best.

Aime: The house thing sounds nice. I'm looking for the camp info and can't find the email. Sarah just told me they have space, though. I'm thinking it's on their website, I'll check.

Lauren: It is open Tues–Sat 10 am–3:30. What works best for you?

Aime: Thursday? Sarah is going to give me the camp stuff at Catherine's lesson Thursday.

Lauren: It does! I'll swing by and pick you up around 10 if that works for you. And thanks for getting camp info. C is really wanting to go.

Aime: That's great. Is it really this way? I'll be fine to drive if it's out of your way! Also–the camp is usually 5 weeks in June and July. I usually sign up for one.

The whole exchange reminded me that Lauren still needed me as a resource as well as a friend, and I was starting to see how I would disappoint her. She didn't seem to grasp what I was going through, and I didn't have the heart to explain it in more detail. Those were the moments when new friendships were tested, and I hoped ours would survive.

I imagined it probably sucked to have one of your first friends in a new place get cancer, but I was quite sure that it was much worse to actually be the one who had it.

CHAPTER 11

Batten Down the Hatches

Dear Friends,

Thank you all for your thoughts and warm wishes to Aime over the last few weeks. The surgery went well and while the tumor was successfully removed, so was a lymph node. She will continue to need your prayers and also some help with meals and playdates, as she begins treatment next week.

We are setting up a schedule on the "Mealtrain" app, which will help organize/calendar what Aime, Scott and the kids' specific needs are. This allows you to review the schedule at your convenience and pick ways in which you can help support them. You'll be receiving an email inviting you to the application in the next day or so. At this time, the needs are most likely to be healthy meals for the family (while mom is resting the kids will definitely need their veggies) and a few playdates. If you don't cook, here are some links to chefs that deliver as well.
https://munchery.com
https://gobble.com

While you will only see April and May populated, we'll be adding to it as Aime's needs change/evolve.

Blessings and many thanks,
Jackie

THE TIME WAS passing rapidly as I approached the start to chemo. I was working as quickly as I was able to get things organized and scheduled to run in my absence. I set up grocery delivery services; hired Judy, an after-school babysitter who could also walk Maverick; and lobbied some friends to write letters to Menlo and Holy Cross for Catherine. There were some things that were slipping through my fingers as I grasped for some semblance of control.

I received a call from the infusion center scheduling my first couple of rounds of chemo, and after we talked briefly about which day of the week would be best, we settled on Wednesdays, and then I looked at the calendar. The first treatment was scheduled on the day of Catherine's drama performance. They were doing Alice in Wonderland and she was the white rabbit.

"Oh," I said, my voice shaking slightly. "Um, that's my daughter's… um, no, I can't start on that day."

The woman on the other end of the line made a sympathetic sound and changed course without hesitation. "Fine, then. We'll do Thursdays. Okay?"

"Yes, thank you." I wiped away a stray tear. How many more moments would I miss? I stood before a great unknown, and while I tried to gather all the information and tools that I could to help, I knew that at a certain point I must walk into the unknown alone.

If I could only get over the hair issue, I thought, running my fingers through my long dark hair, relishing the smooth, shiny strands and the way they curled under just at the ends against my chest. I was preparing myself to say goodbye. Not goodbye, really, just see you later.

Wesley ran his fingers through it at night when I sang his song and said his prayer. Catherine liked to play with it and brush it, pulling it into braids or a side ponytail. Scott sometimes lifted it off my neck when I got hot and blew cool air before he gave my neck a kiss, holding the thick bundle in his hand.

It's only hair, I told myself. But it wasn't really. It was how I knew myself. It was the way I had always been, and I might admit in a more candid moment that it was one of my favorite features. It was how I was described: *You know, the one with the long dark hair.* I couldn't imagine myself without it.

I ran into Rachael, the head of school, at a school coffee one morning. She stopped me and said, "I appreciate how good you are being about this whole process. So many other parents are being so difficult." She was referring to Catherine's middle school applications.

I smiled a bit uneasily in response. "Well, I understand. It's a difficult process. I have to say I have heard that people are holding spots at Holy Cross while waiting for other wait list spots to open up, though, and that does make me a little nervous."

"Oh, don't worry." Her sweet placid face took on a hard edge that took me off guard for an instant. "Those people aren't going *anywhere.*"

I supposed she meant that if they were trying to get into a better school at that point they shouldn't bother. I hoped it didn't mean she would have anything to do with it. It wouldn't help Catherine if they kept their spots anyway.

Oops, I thought. Watch out, Rachael. As we say in the South, your slip is showing.

The next Monday I was on the way to acupuncture, a solid effort to make my immune system as strong as possible, when my phone rang. I put the call on speaker.

"Hello, Aime? It's Rachael Hanlon. Do you have a moment to talk?"

"Oh, hi, Rachael. A minute. What's up?"

"I've just gotten off the phone with Holy Cross. Apparently they have over-subscribed for the first time in twenty-five years, so they are not going into their wait list."

"Over-subscribed?"

"They sent out more acceptances than they had spots for allowing for a certain number of overlap between acceptances from other schools. Normally it works out so that enough people choose other schools and they can go into their wait list, but this year too many people accepted."

"So they're not going into their wait list at all?"

"That's what I've been told. There is always a chance that something changes in the next few months, but as of now, I think we need to look at other options."

"Oh wow. That would have been helpful to start a couple of weeks ago. I am starting chemo this week on Thursday. What other schools are even options at this point?"

"Let me make some calls and I'll see."

"Is there any word from Menlo?"

"I will call and find out. I will let you know as soon as possible."

I hung up the phone, knowing this was going to get a little messy. Crap.

The next morning I asked Shelley and Lauren to meet me at Le Spa. I knew Jackie was out of town, and I trusted Shelley and Lauren to keep me distracted and to offer their immaculate style advice. I had called ahead telling Christian, my stylist, what was going on, but there was a slight language barrier and a significant amount of background noise, and from his reaction I couldn't be sure he had understood me. I had decided to try a short hair style, knowing it was due to fall out within two weeks of starting chemo. Fresh in my mind was Robin Wright's clean style in *House of Cards* with long bangs and a close crop on the back and sides. I'd saved some photos on my phone to show Christian and sat down in the chair, the first to arrive.

"Okay, so I'm ready to do this," I said, my determination exaggerated by my death grip on the arm rests.

"So you want to cut it short?" he asked, picking up a long lock of my hair with his thumb and forefinger while he pumped up the seat.

"Yes, I need to take charge," I said, "I've invited my friends along for support. Oh, here they are!"

Shelley and Lauren came waltzing in all smiles and greetings.

"Did anyone bring some champagne?" Shelley said with her brightest smile. "I thought of it, but I was wondering if it was too early."

"A bit," I said, laughing. "It's 9:55. Look, here are the pictures, you know the woman on *House of Cards*? What do you think?" I held out my phone to Lauren.

"I think it's adorable. You can totally pull it off."

"Yes, completely," Shelley agreed.

"I'm confused, did I miss something?" Christian asked.

"Oh, yes, that's why I called. I'm starting chemotherapy this week, and my hair will all be gone, so I wanted to cut it short in the meantime so there is not so much to lose."

"Oh, I'm sorry, I didn't understand. I'm so sorry. This has been the strangest day. You're the second lady who has asked me to do this. The other one's husband called and asked me to open early this morning."

We all paused, and the girls blinked at him for a moment, unsure what to say.

"Well, do you want me to take a picture of the three of you together?"

"Oh, what a good idea," we all agreed, relieved for the awkwardness to pass.

I got my phone ready to snap the picture and handed it to Christian. We lined up and he smiled at us and snapped a quick shot, then handed my phone back to me. I glanced at the photo on the screen and laughed. It was blurry and Shelley still had her hand up fixing her hair. "It's perfect."

Christian got the girls settled and put my dry hair in a loose ponytail.

"Ok, here we go," he grasped one side of the tail and his sheers sawed through on the inside. It took a few tries before the scissors broke through, making a sickening crunch, crunch, crunch before the ponytail fell away in his hand and my loose hair fell back around my jaw line.

"Oh, Aime, it's so pretty!" Shelley said.

Lauren added, "It highlights your eyes so well."

"You have such a great profile! Look at your graceful neck!" Shelley said.

I laughed as Christian whisked me away to wash my hair. "That's why I brought them."

It started well. I did like the initial shorter length, cropped just below my chin, but I didn't speak up and Christian was determined to be faithful to my wishes and the photos I brought in. So he kept cutting.

The girls and I chatted, but I saw Christian muttering behind me and frowning at my neck. A look and a comment passed between Shelley and Lauren that I missed, and Christian kept cutting shorter and shorter. Slowly a mushroom seemed to appear on top of my head.

I put on my brave face while Christian finished up, and I escaped as quickly as possible. He put my severed ponytail into a little bag and

I walked out with it as if I had bought some hair products. Catherine and Wesley had both said they wanted to keep it, agreeing to split it up between them. But after they held it and played with it a little bit, they never asked for it again. I kept it, though. I still have it in the bag that Christian gave me buried in a basket full of scarves and hats.

We got outside to the courtyard and saw that it had started raining. A light, California rain, but moisture was coming out of the sky nonetheless. We stood for a moment, unsure of what to do.

"Oh, look. There is a pair of doves in the tree. How sweet," Shelley said, looking up.

"Doves!" I cried, as I spotted them huddled against each other, sheltered from the rain under the leaves. "Oh, they always show up for me when I need them."

"My bag!" Shelley startled. "Oh, it stains from the water. I'll be right back." She ran back into the spa, her furry Chanel bag tucked protectively under her arm.

Lauren saw my face and we hurried around the corner, "Aime, it's okay. Just push it down and it just looks like you have a ponytail."

"It's awful!" I broke down. "It's so bad!"

"It's not! It looks fine. It looks nice!" She nodded with determination.

By the time Shelley came back out, I had pulled myself together and we agreed to have lunch at Portola Kitchen. By the time we got there it was pouring rain, the unusual weather seeming to mock my mood. We got settled into a booth and Shelley and Lauren kept up a steady and purposefully lighthearted banter while the entire time I fidgeted with my hair. It felt so strange, so bare, *so someone else*, not me. It was the first moment when I began to see how much my life would change. It rained consistently for the rest of the afternoon.

Lea texted, asking for a photo so I sent it to her.

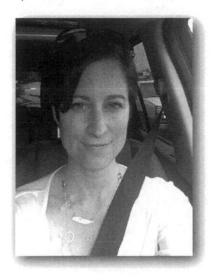

Aime: It's awful.
Lea: Your face ☹ But I love it! Party in the front, business in the back!

I grinned despite myself at the image of a reverse mullet. She was right. It was only temporary. Then Shelley texted later.

Shelley: What did the kids say about the haircut?
Aime: They were fine. Catherine wants to text a pic to her friends—she says it's "text worthy"
Shelley: Haha. One less item of concern. Xo

When Scott got home that night, he did a double take. "Oh that was today?"

"What do you think?" I asked, wrinkling my nose.

"It's good," he said, raising his voice a little. When I looked at him skeptically, he widened his eyes and nodded enthusiastically. "It's good!"

That particular combination of wide eyes with a nod was his "tell," which I never told him I knew.

I started wearing hats around the house then. Scott tried his best to convince me it looked fine, but in a weak moment after a couple of days of trying to be brave, I broke down and cried. "I don't know how you can stand to look at me," I whimpered, knowing it was silly but still feeling like a huge part of myself was missing. My emotions were all wrapped around that major change, and I knew it was only the beginning. What would he think of me when I was bald? What would the kids think? How could I live with myself?

The following day Shelley checked in again.

10:30 a.m.
Shelley: How's your day today?
Aime: Hanging out at Stanford for scans—blech. What are you up to?
Shelley: Have meeting at Village Pub for lunch. Want to meet up this afternoon for tea before you head home?
Shelley: Jim is on the fence about my new emoticon skills (monkey covering eyes)
Shelley: Do they give you drugs there or do you have to wait until you get home?
Aime: I love the new emoticon skills!! It's about time! I'm not sure when I'll be done here. Will text if I have time. The drugs will have to wait until I get home ;)
Shelley: Not fair. If you ever need a driver so you can take drugs in advance, please ask. I am so out and about everywhere from San Carlos to Palo Alto and Los Altos Hills. It would not be a hassle at all. Sending you good thoughts! ☺

1:30 p.m.
Aime: Already done—wasn't as bad as I thought!
Shelley: Nice!
Aime: Starbucks in 20?
Shelley: Meet you there!

Once we secured our favorite corner spot outside, I filled Shelley in quickly about the latest on Catherine's school search and my worries.

"It's such a heavy burden for an eleven-year-old to carry. So many things all at once." I said, welling up into tears. "I didn't think that public school would have to be an option when we moved to San Carlos. We couldn't find anything in Woodside, and I didn't think changing towns would matter that much. I don't know anything about the middle school there. We hardly know anyone in the neighborhood yet, much less with middle schoolers Catherine's age. We don't know anyone whose children go there. The only people who have said anything to me about it at all have talked about how big it is. I think we might need to move. I looked on Craigslist and there are a couple of options. Maybe we could find something on Skyline in Woodside to get back there. Woodside Elementary goes to eighth grade and one of her best friends is going there. I don't know how we're going to manage this, starting a school search from scratch. I start chemo tomorrow! And at this point what schools are going to be available? They all had applications due in January!" I tried to push it down, but the panic was bubbling up beyond my control.

"Well, I hesitate to mention it, but there is this cottage that will be coming up for rent in Woodside." Shelley said. She sat back and locked her electric blue eyes in on me as if she were following a crisis de-escalation check list in her brain. Stay calm. Give the illusion of space while keeping a watchful eye. Offer a solution.

"A cottage?" I looked up, hopeful.

"It's teeny tiny, and I'm not sure if you would even fit, but it's in a fantastic location. The very best in Woodside, and it's on an eight-acre property. Skyline is way too far up the mountain. You need to be closer."

"Eight acres?" I asked, desperately grasping at straws and imagining Maverick romping along outside and the kids roaming free. "What do you mean by teeny tiny?"

Shelley pulled her lips back into a tight smile while she tilted her head, her blonde hair cascading to her shoulders. "Small. I think it's about fourteen hundred square feet. But it's really very sweet. And the land. There is something almost magical about it." She looked up toward the blue sky dotted with a few wispy clouds. "And honestly, I think you really are just a better fit in Woodside. I think it's time to get your family back there, and then Catherine's schooling will be all taken care of."

"I agree, I'm a country girl. Maybe it's my Nashville roots, but I can't help it. I need some open air and trees or I start going crazy." I pulled my puffy down jacket around my shoulders and crossed my legs, noticing the contrast between my brown leather riding boots with jeans and Shelley's black heels, probably Prada, and slacks. That pretty much summed it up. Our styles, our personalities.

"Yes, I would say you are definitely Woodside or Portola Valley. Sorry, it's an occupational hazard for a real estate agent to typecast people into neighborhoods. It's okay, because I know I am Menlo Park. Jim thinks we could be Woodside, but I don't see it. Maybe certain parts. But you have that polished, Jackie O, East Coaster thing going but with an earthy blend. Woodside. I am just a fancy lady. Menlo Park."

I laughed at her use of the term earthy. I knew women I considered earthy who would roll their eyes at my makeup and jewelry. Shelley probably just thought I was earthy because I preferred flip flops and maxi skirts in the summer over heels. "I think you nailed it. So how are things going with the girls? I haven't been able to catch up with anyone else in a while."

"Well, everyone is spending a lot of time trying to find the best ways we can help you."

"Translation?" I asked, picking up my drink and poking the straw deeper into the ice to reach the last few sips of tea.

"There might be a few disagreements as to what you need versus what you are saying you need."

"Coming from?"

"I don't know. Only people that love you very much."

"That's so sweet for everyone to worry. I'll just be honest with you. I only need what I am asking for. I can't think of anything else. If something new comes up, I promise I will let you know!"

"And I just want to throw it out there that the benefit will still be an option for you if you decide you want to go at the last minute."

"Yeah, thanks. It's really sweet, but I'm pretty sure I won't feel like going. With the benefit being on Saturday, and my treatment tomorrow, it falls at the worst possible time. I will probably be feeling pretty bad that day."

"Okay, I'm just going to hold you a seat just in case." She nodded at me as if to change my decision, and I shook my head.

"Team Aime" had such good intentions. Everything they did for me was out of love, and I knew it and felt it. But so many of the suggestions they made highlighted to me how little they really understood what I was going through. I didn't want to go on to them about how bad it was and would get, but I didn't want to go to the fucking benefit either. I couldn't have cared less about the benefit.

The Starbucks run put me off my timing, and I had to hurry to pick up Wesley in time. Catherine was already at riding, and I had just enough time to scoop Wesley up before heading to the barn. I pulled quickly into the school parking lot, rushing past the office toward the main outdoor staircase that led to the aftercare classroom. One of the administrators sauntered toward me and I put my guard up, knowing she would be thinking about Catherine's middle school situation, or at least should be. She had sat in the meeting that past fall nodding in agreement as I asked if we were okay applying to just two schools. She was also the one I asked about the test prep classes that everyone else seemed to be doing in the fall. She had told me she didn't think it would be necessary for Catherine because "sometimes these efforts backfire and make the children nervous instead of being helpful." I pulled my features back into a tight polite smile, and she said hello in return.

Then she stopped, turning, and exclaimed, "Oh, you cut your hair!"

Fuck, I'd almost forgotten. "Yes," I said, smoothing down the thick poof self-consciously.

"Oh, what a shame! I mean, it's cute, of course, but I always admired your beautiful, long hair the way it curled just perfectly and flowed out behind..." She went on gesturing bodily with her hands shaking out her own great head as if imaginary locks flowed behind. "Oh well," she sighed and turned back toward the office.

I continued on toward the staircase. My knees weakened a little, and I tried to hide my urge to vomit as the bile rose in my throat. Rachael said she had told her. What was going on? Apparently she didn't know, or had forgotten, why I had let my luscious locks go. *It's because I have cancer, you fucking cow.*

Later that night Scott and I talked over the idea of moving. We agreed. It was something we could and should consider. I texted Shelley to let her know.

Aime: Scott is open to the moving to Woodside idea—I'm falling in love with the cottage idea—cozy!

Shelley: I will have the key on Monday. Let's plan to see Tuesday after drop off? Or whatever time works for you. It's small. But you will be the very first to see it.

Aime: I can see it Tuesday but I'm not sure if I can drive by then. When will it be available?

Shelley: We can figure out. I can always pick you up. Ha keep you all day to hang out with me...

Aime: You could pick us all up on the way to school and keep me with you ☺

Shelley: Ok! I will plan on picking you up Tuesday morning ☺

Aime: Yay! I love real estate ☺

Shelley: Me too! Most days...

Shelley: What is your schedule tomorrow? How does the day work? Is there anywhere we can assist or be available? Xo

Aime: I've got tests and appointments all morning then if everything is clear, which so far it has been, we start chemo at 12:30 and it lasts till 4:30. I think it will be fine! Scott will be there with me the whole time. You've done so much already (hearts)

Shelley: Ok. Get some rest tonight. Know how much we all love you. My candle is lit right now sending positive thoughts and energy. I am in Redwood City, Palo Alto and Menlo Park tomorrow and available to assist with kids, etc. if needed. Xo

Aime: xoxoxo

CHAPTER 12

Letter to Chemo
April—Week One

THERE HAD BEEN a lot of anxiety building up to that moment, but by Thursday there I was, sitting in the carefully decorated waiting room, having just had my port accessed for the first time. I can't describe the process as anything other than creepy. It's not particularly painful, but knowing there is a plastic cup just under the skin with a tube leading up to and into my jugular is a weird feeling. The nurse had chatted casually with me while I sat in the chair watching her every move. She pulled out a package of materials consisting of alcohol wipes, sterile gloves and gauze, a large, marble-sized square cup attached to a drain, and an assortment of vials and syringes. She wiped the area clean, held the little suction cup, which upon closer inspection I noticed had a rather large needle in the middle, and placed it directly over the bump which was the port on the right side of my chest about three inches under my clavicle.

"One, two, take a breath," I breathed in deeply as she said, "three" and pressed hard on the piece. I felt a dull pain accompanied by a sharp pinch, and then it was in. The nurse attached a syringe, explaining, "Now I have to flush the port." She pulled the stopper out a little, and blood rushed into the chamber. "That's good. It's how we know it's in right," she said. She pushed the stopper back in fully, and I immediately tasted the saline in the back of my nose. It reminded me of playing in overly chlorinated pools as a child and getting water up my nose after a bad flip. I felt a chill through my veins as the cool liquid flooded in.

After I was thoroughly flushed, she filled three vials with blood at an alarmingly quick pace, then she put a cap on the port access device and taped the whole thing to my chest, explaining that I would need to leave it on for the infusion later, "so we don't have to poke you twice," she said with a smile.

"No, we don't want that," I said.

She directed me to the office area to check in for my appointment with Dr. S, the oncologist. I knew it would be a little while before they got the results and before I could meet with the doctor, but I didn't have time to go anywhere else, so I chose to camp out in the waiting room.

I had already had time to become familiar with the cancer center in a way one hopes never to have to, and though I knew the rooms were carefully contrived in a way to appear peaceful, I appreciated the effort because the effect was more soothing than your average hospital clinic.

The room was sectioned into four pod areas separated by wood and frosted glass, and each area was lined with an assortment of chairs and sectional sofas all in neutral earth tones. The walls were painted a warm camel color with a hint of rose, and in addition to soft overhead lighting, corner table lamps lent the room a comfortable living room atmosphere. A couple of flat screen TVs ran slides advertising programs at Stanford and the news, and there were magazines, informational pamphlets and tissue boxes scattered around. All of this was designed to provide a neutral support to whatever emotion erupted from the expected range of boredom, grief, anxiety, and irritation to a sort of cheerful camaraderie that often occurred between patients.

A text popped up on my phone from Lauren.

Lauren: Thinking of you. You are stronger than you think, braver than anyone I know and loved. Xoxo

After some time I was called back into the clinic. A nurse checked my vitals and left me to change and wait some more. Dr. S came in announcing that my blood test looked good and we were all set to go. She gave me a little pep talk and answered a few questions, then patted me on the knee. "Okay, then. Let's do this."

I walked out of the building and crossed the street to the infusion center. A text from Scott popped up asking where I was so he could meet me. I had asked him to wait until the infusion to meet me because I knew that would be the time I needed him most. Already we were being cautious about the amount of time he would be able to take from work and wanted to use it most effectively.

I gave my name and birthdate to a very friendly receptionist, and she motioned for me to sit in another waiting area. Scott rushed in and sat next to me, fiddling with his briefcase. "How did everything go with Dr. S?"

"It was fine. My blood test looked good. Everything is proceeding according to plan," I said, my best "everything is fine" assurance.

"That's good. Did you get lunch yet?" He shifted around in his seat, trying to get comfortable in the chairs that were clearly not meant for his 6'2", 240-lb frame.

"No, I hadn't thought about it." My stomach was in knots already.

"That's okay, once you get started I might head down to the deli and get some snacks for us."

"That's a good idea. I could probably use some water, too."

Then a nurse came into the waiting room and called my name.

"Here we go," I whispered as we walked over to greet her.

"Hi Aime, my name is Sarah. I'm going to be your nurse today. Have you had your vitals checked already?"

"Yes, at the clinic."

"Great. So we're going to be in section C." She led me down a long corridor past sections A and B, and I got my first glance at what the rooms looked like. Each section was the size of the main waiting room and was set up with four private rooms on the side and an open area with a wall of windows in which there were about eight infusion stations. Each station had a large reclining chair, curtains that could be pulled around for privacy, and a flat screen TV on a huge metal arm that could be pulled in front of the chair or pushed away. A cushioned bench stretched along below the entire length of windows, and there were floating chairs for visitors placed sporadically around the room.

She led me into a station that was tucked into a corner of the interior wall next to the doorway that led to section D. "Is this okay?" she asked as if she were a hostess seating me in a restaurant.

"I guess so. It's my first time today, so I don't really know what it's going to be like."

"Oh, it's your first time? You'll do fine." She assured me.

"Do you have a chair for Scott?" I asked while I settled into the reclining chair and began fiddling with the controls.

"Oh yes, I'll be right back with that and some warm blankets. Anything else you need?"

"Not right now, thanks."

Scott and I looked at each other blankly. I moved my legs and gestured for him to sit with me while we waited. The anticipation was getting to us both. He sat down near my feet with his back towards me. It was the only way he would fit on the chair. My hand went distractedly and automatically to run my fingernails over his back. The feel of his broad shoulders under my fingertips making me feel more secure.

Scott kept his hair cropped close to his head. I loved it when he let it grow a little longer in the summers, but he would complain about it getting itchy and ask me to run my fingers through it, scratching his scalp gently at night before he slept. He was a gentle giant, his tall frame towering over me and his arm span wrapping easily around me. He had kind blue eyes, a prominent forehead and a strong nose that would seem too big on another face, but somehow added a distinguished look to his. He was ruggedly handsome in a way that was reminiscent of an ancient Roman gladiator, but he kept clothed in rumpled

Brooks Brothers and North Face jackets. His shoulders hunched slightly from countless hours over decades in front of the computer, and he wore wire and tortoise-framed glasses as a result of the corresponding eye strain. He reminded me of Clark Kent before the transformation. I knew Super Man was under there somewhere.

The nurse came right back and started to explain how the process would work. "Okay, I've put in the order with the pharmacy for your meds. I'll start to access your port now, then we start with a drip of Pepcid and Decadron to help you manage the chemo better. That will take about thirty minutes to take effect. And then we start the chemotherapy."

"Oh, okay," I said.

Scott settled in beside me, and the nurse bustled around flushing my port and setting up the IV. I spent the next half hour fussing around in my bag while Scott banged out some emails. I had read a chemo checklist that offered ideas of what to bring along, and I had followed the suggestion to the letter: Book, movie loaded on my tablet, magazines, fully charged phone, charger as a backup, ginger chews for nausea, mints to help with the saline taste from the flushing, shawl. I pulled the shawl out, wrapping it around me even though I wasn't yet cold. My friend Debbie from Boston had sent it to me for the occasion, and wrapping it around me felt like she was giving me a warm hug.

The nurse bustled back to my station. "Okay, I have the order from the pharmacy. So we can go ahead and get started." She had suited up in protective gear from head to toe to prevent any of the medicine from touching her skin. The medicine itself was labeled with a huge yellow sticker on the side proclaiming "Caution! Contains highly toxic material," which would in just a few moments be seeping into my body. She placed two gigantic syringes the size of an extra-large tube of toothpaste filled with what looked like red fruit punch on the side table. "This I have to push into your IV by hand."

She attached the syringe to my IV and sat down beside me, holding it carefully between her gloved hands. She had also placed a plastic apron over her scrubs and a mask over her face. This must be the much-maligned red devil, I thought. I had heard all about it on the cancer message boards. Otherwise known as Red Death, it is so toxic that only a certain small measure of doses can be given to a person over the span of her entire life, and it is known to cause permanent side effects, including heart disease and neuropathy among a battery of other problems. I looked again at the large yellow label on the side of the syringe warning: TOXIC. No kidding.

I leaned my head back against the cool gray leather of the chair and took a deep breath. So far, so good. Nothing major had happened. I remembered the advice the naturopath had given me: to imagine the chemo coming into my body as little fairies who know just where to go and what to do without causing any extra damage. I thought about it for a moment and figuring it couldn't hurt, I offered a prayer.

The nurse finished the Adriamycin push and hooked up the Cytoxan drip. "Now we just let this work for about ninety minutes and we're done. I'll come back to check on you in a few. Just push that red call button if you need anything. Okay?"

"Thanks," I muttered and Scott stood up to let her by.

He sat back down next to me. "You doing okay?"

"Yeah, it's fine." I sighed and shrugged my shoulders.

We passed the rest of the time mostly silent. It was such an odd feeling, my body filling up with bags and syringes of heavy drugs while I sat still waiting for the effects to hit. For the other shoe to drop.

We went home and Judy, our new sitter, greeted us at the door. The kids were happy, fed, and peacefully doing their homework. I gave them each a hug and kiss and went to bed, jotting out a quick note on an online journal called CareZone I had started to let my friends and family all know how I was doing and to track my progress.

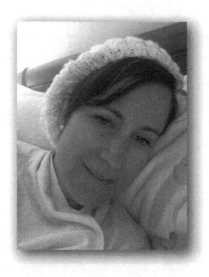

A letter to chemo: I welcome you into my body graciously. I know you are a powerful agent and can make me well again. Combined with healing energy and prayers you are at your highest and most clear power. At this point you have free reign to travel through all the little hidden spots in my body. You are easily able to find any cancer cells that might be lingering or thinking of forming and you can eliminate them. They've served their purpose, I am learning my lessons and it's time for them to move on. Chemo, because you are so strong and clear you can see the difference between cells that are harmful for me and those to leave alone. You may work in this way and I trust you to do your job exceedingly well and I thank you for it.*

*I was under the influence of a huge amount
of medication when that was written

I felt full, almost water logged, and sluggish as if all of the fluid pumped into my body had wrapped me in a liquid bubble. I sighed heavily as I fumbled with the bottle cap for my Ativan. I kept notes on my phone to keep track of all of the drugs—Zofran and Compazine to tamp down the nausea, Hydrocodone for the pain, Decadron to minimize allergic reactions and give my body a fighting boost, and last but not least, Ativan to make it all seem okay. Up until this all started, the strongest thing I had ever taken on a regular basis was Advil.

The combination must have been right because I passed the night fine. I woke up feeling numb and shaky, but I couldn't tolerate the thought of food. Scott and the kids didn't wake me in the morning, and I had a vague memory of Scott lifting the blanket and peering in at me to whisper goodbye as they left. I got up sometime mid-morning and had a quick shower, then climbed back into bed before I regained the energy to get dressed and made up.

Judy brought me back to the hospital for my booster shot, and I typed out a cheerful message to my family and the girls letting them know I was okay.

Then Lauren checked in:

Lauren: How's it today? Watching Wesley and James get excited for their playdate. Smiling faces abound ☺ Ps. Your journal is beautiful. You are amazing and so strong. Hope booster went well. Xox
Aime: Oh good! Glad the boys are happy! Booster was easy, we'll see how I take it. Some people don't even really feel it much, so I'm hoping to be in that bunch! And please excuse all the selfies on the journal! It's for the benefit of my family to see that I'm fine ☺
Lauren: No I love it. It helps me to know you're fine too :)

The replies of encouragement flooded my inbox along with a note from Rachael, who was resorting to email as the news on the middle school front had gotten worse and worse. Menlo was full. She said she would scramble to reach out to alternate schools for Catherine. Great. I didn't even have the words to respond and shot a quick response to Scott: "Can you take this one?" Shit.

Saturday passed in a foggy haze. The room darkened with the late winter sky outside, and I stayed buried under my blankets in bed late into the day, staring blankly out the window where I watched a squirrel scamper back and forth on the branches of the closest water oak. My attention drifted to the curtains framing the large picture window, probably hung by that cute young couple we were sub-leasing the home from. They looked new, most likely ready-made panels from Target or somewhere, but they were woven on the rod the wrong way so that the liner showed on the end. It would be good to fix that someday, I thought, but didn't move to make a note on my phone the way I usually would. I just stared at it for a while, then out at the tree again, and then I closed my eyes exhausted from the effort of thought.

Intermittently throughout the day I woke with what I later came to identify as bone pain—a crushing weight on my sternum and rotating, sharp aches through my large bones and joints. My stomach felt like a pile of rocks.

I thought briefly about my friends at the benefit. Last year I had taken great care getting ready for the night, having my hair, nails, makeup and even lashes done before I stepped into a new dress for the occasion.

I was falling asleep when my phone started lighting up with texts. I fumbled around for it on the bedside table, then pulled it under the covers. I peered through blurry eyes to see that Lauren had sent me a photo. It was of Catherine looking peacefully into the camera with a quiet smile on her face projected on a big screen at the benefit with the caption: "At the beginning of third grade, I was a very shy person, who was afraid to go to a new school. I was afraid of being left out and forgotten. Weeks went by, and I became less shy every one of those weeks. Soon I was confident to face the world and meet new people. To me, this school has such a positive energy, and that's what I most love about Episcopal School."

Shelley: When we saw Catherine's photo we all cried and gave Rachael dirty looks
Jackie: We miss you! Love you tons!

As I drifted off, in my mind I thought about the women who had worked so long to make the benefit happen—all the meetings and calls and hours spent soliciting and organizing donations not to mention the time it took to plan the party itself and secure the food, wine, and decor. I hoped they were all having a wonderful time, and as I laid my head down on my pillow and fell into oblivion, I was glad I wasn't there. In fact, I never wanted to waste my time that way again.

On Sunday I shuffled into the kitchen a little winded from the effort but feeling vaguely hungry and knowing a little food would give me some energy at least. I pulled out a pan for eggs and the weight of it was too much. It dropped to the floor. A cloud fell over me. The eggs, the oil, the spatula—suddenly it felt like an insurmountable task. Then even the thought of opening the refrigerator turned my stomach. I couldn't do it. Scott came up behind me, and I turned into his big chest and cried. My fingers touched the soft flannel of his shirt, and I breathed in the familiar musky mix of Old Spice deodorant and Ivory soap.

"I didn't think it would last this long," I whispered against his chest.

"Well, okay," he said in a "we can make it one more mile" kind of voice. "It's Sunday, so it should be going away soon. It'll go away." He rubbed my back and kissed the top of my head.

"I think we're going to need to move again."

"For Catherine?" he asked, and I nodded in response.

"Shhh," he breathed in my hair. "Don't worry about that now. We'll figure it out."

I charted the rest of the days in notes on my phone:

Day 4 started to see hints of getting better but took a while
Day 5 mellow day – sluggish – improving

I was starting to come out of the fog, but my brain still felt mushy and confused. After I spent a couple of hours staring out the window again from my bed, I sat up, trying to shake it off. I wanted to check back in with Laura, the survivor I had been emailing with. I lamented that she hadn't worked out as a sitter, but her correspondence had become invaluable to me.

To: Laura Z
From: Aime Card
Subject: Checking in

Hi Laura,

Day 5. That was a doozy! I wasn't prepared for the head fog. I knew about it, but wow. I'm still just sort of sitting in my bed confused as to what to do today. Yikes!
How long did it take you to bounce back? Do you ever really bounce back during chemo? I just keep imagining myself jumping up and down at the end of all this, relishing in my strength again, but it's sometimes hard to imagine it coming back all the way.
I think I'm trying to borrow some of your rock star attitude!

Aime

To: Aime Card
From: Laura Z
Subject: Re: Checking in
GET OUT THE WEED!!!

Remember I said my husband would have to remind me?
I'm reminding you.
Then see how you feel. I only ever take one hit. Don't want to crossover into paranoia...Lol
If you are wide awake?

Put on some great music, cozy clothes, light some candles and clean, organize, plant flowers etc. to keep yourself busy.
Yet all the time knowing you can get back in bed if necessary.
My side of the bed was command central.

Do you have a TV in your room? If not make command central on the couch. That way you can be in the mix and shout orders at everyone... And kids can come snuggle whenever they want for as long as they want.

So I lived under the covers reading, and watching movies, and when I got antsy I cleaned. (Then I got to feel so good hiding under the covers knowing everything was in order instead of beating myself up that my house is getting out of control)

Also, make easy recipe cookies or food you don't normally have the time to do and the kids will be excited when they get home.
Worst case scenario is you have to stop and get back under the covers right?
So what if you leave a mess somewhere. You are just always doing your best and everyone knows that.

So get in the right frame of mind to prepare yourself for not having one... Ha ha ha!!

Yesterday I told my daughter in Michigan, I am so embarrassed I could cry.
Please tell me what degree you will have in June again? I need to tattoo it on my wrist because it is GONE from my brain and refuses to stay after someone tells me.
Our daughter in Chicago?

People ask what her major is and I say she's getting her masters in Hockey. (She plays university hockey as well)
I can't EFFing remember!!!

So, lol
It will get better than it actually "feels" now but it is a gift that keeps on giving.

My mom died from breast cancer at 52. She chose not to do chemo. Only radiation. So I figure I'd rather be here for my kids with brain fog than not be here at all. Right?
Perspective!!

DRINK WATER!
I could barely make myself do it and wish I'd done more
During the actual chemo process.
This poison is going through your entire system and attacking every cell.
Good news is we make new ones. But the brain is something I didn't think about at the time. So flood your body with water, organic soup broths, teas to carry the residue out.

That is one regret I have, and also that I didn't get out in the sunshine and walk.

I'm off to an interview.

Smoke some dope! If you need me to pick you up the perfect little tiny pipe that closes up and hides easily let me know. I will go buy one for you. I think they are around 25.00. You can stay stoned the whole time if it makes you feel better. Why not?

You're going to be bald and have bloodshot eyes anyway — Might as well giggle through it.

If you use Pandora, get the
"Madeleine Peyroux" station or "Norah Mercer" and turn it up! You are on vacation!

Talk soon, stay strong!
(((HUGS)))

To: Laura Z
From: Aime Card
Subject: Re: Checking in

Lol!!!!! You are the absolute best! That is exactly what I needed to hear!

Also, I'm sorry about your mom. My mom passed away last year with a brain tumor. She had breast cancer about 7 years before and only had radiation. I wonder if she'd had chemo if it would have prevented the brain tumor. It's extra motivation to stick around for the kids. I know how much they need me. I think you must be an angel that came into my life at just the right time. ok – mushy chemo brain!!

To: Aime Card
From: Laura Z
Subject: Re: Checking in

I am so blown away by the similarity of our stories and I am soooo sorry to hear you lost your mother so recently. I know too well how it hurts so effing bad!

Worst for me was my daughter not having her around.
But they are with us, life goes on and kids do just fine.

So keep me posted!

Knowing that Laura had gone through this with grace and laughter just a couple of years before boosted my spirits enough to help me pull through the following few days. It wasn't until after the next round that I understood why the doctors had kept warning about talking to others about their experiences. "Every experience is different," they had said, and I should have listened better. At that point I was just happy to hear someone else laughing in the face of it.

I smoked some dope, like Laura suggested, but it wasn't doing much for me. I imagined it was because I was so loaded up with other chemicals. But I did like the rebellious feeling it gave me. It made me feel like I could still make some of my own choices and take back some kind of control.

Then I moved through the days and climbed back toward myself taking notes to track my progress.

Days 6–11 gradually able to get out and maintain a small version of my life
Days 12–13 really almost normal, but would crash in the evening after a normal day of running around. A scrape on my finger refused to heal—used antibiotic ointment daily with very slow healing, then tried Manuka honey, which helped dramatically. Some aches and pains here and there—took Ibuprofen, neck discomfort—slight soreness in mouth—have swished with coconut oil the last two mornings and seems to help.

CHAPTER 13

The Cottage
Week Two

Shelley: Good morning. How are you? Can I still pick you and kids up tomorrow?

Aime: It works for us!

Shelley: Ok good. Thinking Abby and I will pick you guys up a little after 7:30? Then we will go see rental. I can take you home at some point, (hehe)

Shelley:

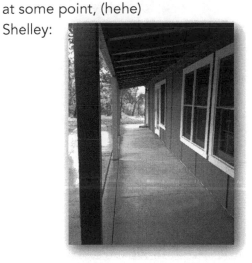

Aime: It looks really sweet! Do you think there is room for a king in the MBR?

Shelley: Yes but nothing else ☺

Aime: even a chest? Is the closet decent?

Shelley: Lots of closet and drawers.

Aime: Oh, perfect! I'm tired of the old New England dresser anyway!

Shelley: Lol, that's just half the wall. Only Woodside?

Aime: It's preferred.

Shelley: Let's check it out tomorrow and you can decide.

Aime: I think small is not so bad. Do you think more than one bed will fit in the other br? Or would it need to be bunked?

Shelley: No. could be two beds.

Aime: You're right. We can see then!

Shelley: You can even do a bunk bed with homework space underneath. That might be neat for Wesley. And Catherine could have the other side of the room.

Aime: Yes, that's a good idea. IKEA is made for small spaces!!

Shelley: Thing about the cottage is the setting is amazing, the location is the best and there is a fenced area for Mav so that makes me feel a bit better for the overall fit. I will see what else I can come up with over the next couple of weeks.

Aime: I am feeling good about this one. The living room looks pretty big and for sleeping we can be cozy ☺

SHELLEY DROVE INTO Woodside and made a left on Mountain Home Road at the intersection across from Roberts Market. I hadn't been back since we'd moved to San Carlos the previous summer, and I'd forgotten how much I loved the town. Just on the other side of the 280, the hustle and bustle of Silicon Valley settled right down and the area felt authentically rural. The main buildings in town retained an old frontier look nestled into ancient redwoods, bay trees, and water oaks. We crossed the two little stone bridges and turned left onto Manzanita Way, which was marked by a massive bay tree with at least a ten-foot-wide whitewashed-looking trunk with the strips of bark peeling down onto the mulched horse path below. The little street wound around under a latticework of arched tree limbs with sunlight filtering through. We pulled into a gravel driveway with an old farm gate. Shelley got out and pushed back the gate, letting it drag a little across the stones.

The gravel turned to pavement about halfway up the driveway, and we pulled up in front of a small ranch style cottage nestled between the trees on a slight ridge with a view of the mountain rising up in the distance behind. This was the style for which the popular sixties architecture had been named, the cottage easily predating the suburban sprawl.

"Here we are," Shelley said as we got out of the car. My gaze roved over the spread of open land that was so rare in the area. The owners had kept the land cleared in the graceful spacing of at least forty ancient water oaks. The smell of bay leaves and eucalyptus filled the air from recent tree trimming and a gentle breeze wafted up over the slope on the other side of the house as if in greeting.

"It's perfect."

"Don't you want to see inside?" Shelley asked, teasing a little.

"Absolutely."

Inside I was charmed by the dark wood beams on the open ceiling and the brick fireplace that stretched almost across the entire end of the main room. The cottage was in impeccable condition. It had obviously been well cared for over the years. It would be a welcome change from our previous two rentals, which remained in a constant state of disrepair, typical for the kind of rental in the area that would accept children and especially pets. I paced out the rooms, immediately visualizing where our furniture would fit. Half would probably go to storage, but I liked the idea of streamlining our belongings.

"Shelley, I think it can really work. Don't you? What do we need to do to get it?"

"Let me see what I can do."

Suddenly everything seemed to fall into place. A school for Catherine; a fantastic yard for the kids, Maverick, and Pluto the cat; a ten-minute drive to Stanford instead of thirty; and we could all be back in this neighborhood that we loved. Finally, something seemed to be going our way.

That afternoon, I texted Shelley.

> Aime: Scott closed his deal!! And he says if I like the house he's happy, so we don't have to wait for him to see it. He's fine with the May 1st start.
> Shelley: That's fantastic. Congrats to Scott. I will send you the application.

Two days later the lease was signed and we officially called off the school search. Later Shelley admitted to me that she had asked her client, the owner of the property, for a favor for the first time in her career. She didn't want to put the listing on the open market, which could have resulted in multiple offers and bidding wars. It was what usually happened with a place like that, and she just wanted us to have it.

The next day I called Sarah Park. Her daughter, Claire, was a close friend of Catherine's and she had made the decision early in the year to pull both her daughters out of Episcopal and send them to Woodside Elementary the following year. They were the only family in Catherine's class who had chosen to skip the independent middle school application process altogether in favor of public school. I wanted to let her know our news and was interested to hear her opinion.

Sarah was a straight talker, and I knew she would have something good to say.

"Aime, how is everything going? How are you doing?"

120

"I'm okay, I've made it through the first round."

"That's great. You know, I said to Scott the other day, and I'll say it again to you. I know it's a pain to have to go through, but I know you can get through it. I've had several friends lately that have had to deal with similar things. The treatment has come so far now. Before we used to hear about people catching it late with only so long to live, but now it's more about just having to live through the treatment."

"You know, you're right. Scott mentioned that he appreciated you said that. He's had to run interference for me with so many people with panicked concerns that it was refreshing to him to have your support and your calm attitude."

"Well, just let me know as always if there is anything we can do."

I filled her in on the school update and our plans to move.

"You're going to love Woodside Elementary," she assured me. "There are going to be just thirty-five kids in their entire grade this year. I've been so impressed with their program. Claire has met some of the girls already, and they seem really sweet. They're also excited about new girls joining the class."

After we talked for a minute about how glad the girls would be to go to school together, the conversation switched gears.

"You know this looks terrible for Episcopal. Once people find out that you had to move your family to go to a public school, the shockwaves are going to be massive. It's not what Episcopal advertises, and it's not what the families expect. I don't mean to add fuel to the fire, but the word around Episcopal is that Rachael might have made a mistake here," Sarah said.

"I've been wondering about that. I saw her at carpool yesterday and she had this terribly, almost comically, guilty look on her face when she saw my car. I wondered what the hell she had to feel guilty about," I said.

"Some people have suggested that with one of the schools she puts in special requests for particular students, you know, her special projects. She must have assumed that Catherine would be fine since she is such a good student, and when she was waitlisted, Rachael had to scramble. Initially she probably didn't think you would get so many people upset on your behalf, being new to the school, but now that everyone knows what else you are dealing with, they are so angry for you. The fact that she was not able to help Catherine off the wait list just shows everyone what little influence she really has at the end of the day. I guess if you're not one of the people she pushes for, and who knows how you make that list, you're out of luck."

"So not only was Catherine in line behind siblings, Portola Valley residents, alumni, and friends of board members but behind particular choices of Rachael's too? It kind of makes you wonder about the priorities of the school in general. It's weird. I mean, I just feel so blindsided by the whole process. If we had just had a warning, you know? If we had had some challenge with Catherine, or some indication that we needed to cast a broad net, it would have been different, but there was nothing. She's never gotten a B, she had great test scores, her teachers love her. I don't get it."

"Yeah. Nobody does. At any rate, it'll be great to have you guys back in Woodside. And Claire will be so excited that she and Catherine will both be at Woodside El. So maybe in the end it will all be fine. I'm just sorry you had to go through all of this in the process."

"Yeah, thanks. Me too."

We said our good-byes and I hung up the phone. I sat immobile on the couch, reeling from the implications of all we had said. It was becoming clear to me that while Rachael did make a handful of calls trying to help Catherine after she was wait-listed, that was her job. She should have been doing it before the decisions were made, and not just for her favorites.

And while I knew I would be angry later, at that moment I only felt sorry for her. She was caught off guard. She was a little checked out, doing things the way she had for the previous decades, another casualty of the beast that Silicon Valley had become. Adapt or die, progress at the speed of light or be left behind. I wondered if we would survive it, or if we should run for the hills, back to a place where things made sense.

Jackie had agreed to meet me later at the wig shop. It was not a task I wanted to take on alone. She was already there when I walked in, sitting on the little bench in reception. I gave her a hug, then made a face, sucking air through my teeth.

She laughed and gave me a quick kiss on the cheek, her hands resting on my forearms. We had the habit of glancing over each other's outfits when we first said hello, always finding something to compliment. It was an old habit I supposed we both shared from growing up with sisters.

"You look pretty," I said.

"So do you. I love this jacket on you," Jackie said.

While Shelley was all about the labels, Jackie kept a much more classic look but no less flattering. She was always proud to inform me of a great deal at Nordstrom Rack or that her dress was five years old. She worked hard for her money and she did not waste a dime.

"Okay." She let out a long breath. "Are you ready for this?" She nodded and looked closely at my reaction, as if coaching or at least coaxing me to be positive about this.

"Yeah, let's see what this is all about," I said as we followed the stylist back to a private room. I had already gotten a preview of how the service would work with the chilly conversation I had had on the phone while making the appointment. Maybe it was just the stylist's lack of personality, but it seemed to me like a gentle touch when dealing with people at a hair replacement salon would be a good business strategy. Or maybe they just felt like people were there out of desperation, so it didn't matter how they behaved. For whatever reason, the stylist was abrupt.

She gestured to a chair in front of a mirror. "So you're looking for a wig?"

"Yes, I'm going through chemotherapy now, and I've been told I have a little over a week left before it starts to really fall out. It's thinning already."

"Yes," she said in a flat tone. "So what length were you thinking of? You mentioned short on the phone, so I pulled out a few along with some medium lengths just to have a variety." She started pulling down Styrofoam head forms from the shelves with a variety of wigs attached to them by long silver hat pins, giving the heads an odd look as if they were once live animals that had been pinned up for dissection.

She put a couple of short wigs on me, and Jackie and I immediately agreed they were just weird looking. I had thought with my short haircut if I had a short wig it would blend in a little better, and my hair wouldn't have so far to grow back to feel normal after my treatment. But the strategy did not hold out, and if I had to wear a wig for however long, I might as well like it.

"These aren't working. Can we try some of the mid-length styles?" I asked. Without meaning to, I had begun to mirror her brusque manner.

She brought down a couple of good options, and I started warming to the idea. Already sick of my new cut, it was nice to play with some longer hair.

"That looks nice," Jackie nodded enthusiastically at a layered wig that fell in soft locks around my face, "and the color is good, too. I like the red tone on you."

"Maybe," I paused frowning at my expression. "So how much is this one?" I asked. I tilted my head back and forth, trying to get comfortable with it.

"That one is $1200. It's real human hair. The synthetic wigs will run a little less, more in the $700–800 range," she said.

Jackie and I widened our eyes at each other. I hadn't expected them to be that costly. For that price I'd rather buy a new piece of furniture.

"Wow, that's more than I expected," I said. "Do you have other options? Are there any used ones or anything?"

She sniffed. "We don't have used ones for hygienic purposes. You would have to go to a charity or somewhere like that."

I smarted at her attitude and let out a long breath. At least I could afford it, even though it added insult to a very bad injury to have to shell out that kind of money for something decidedly un-fun. But what about all the other women who couldn't? Would they be given the same attitude and forced to walk out the door empty-handed as well as bald headed? It was devastating to even think about.

I decided to let it go for the sake of moving on and said, "Well, okay. Let's try on a few more options—and focus on the synthetic ones."

I tried several more in a range of styles and colors, but I kept going back to the $1200 one. It just seemed the most natural, like me with a haircut, not me being some other person, and I liked it a heck of a lot better than the mushroom I was currently walking around with, although as a side note, the thinning of my hair did make it lay a little more nicely for that brief moment in time.

"All right, how does the process work?" I asked, back in my favorite wig again.

The stylist perked up a little, sensing the possibility of an imminent sale. "Well, the cost is really a package deal. It includes your first style and shaving of your head. Once you give us a deposit, we can have it ready for you within a couple of days."

I blinked a little at the head-shaving comment. "I don't know. It's a lot of money for just a short time. I mean, I may only be wearing it for three or four months. My team said I would start growing hair back once I start Taxol in a few weeks."

"Oh, no. You'll be wearing a wig for at least the next year and a half," the stylist said.·

"What? No, my hair grows really fast. I'm sure it won't take that long. No one has suggested it would take that long at all." I argued with her. It didn't help that I already disliked her.

"It's going to take a really long time. I know. I see it every day," she said, folding her arms across her chest.

"Well, maybe for other people." I replied as I stared back at her through the mirror, my back still turned in her direction.

Jackie watched the exchange with a tight smile and diplomatically interjected, "Could you give us a minute, please? It would probably help if we talked it out a little, don't you think?" She nodded at me quickly, then leveled a steady gaze at the woman until she left the room.

"Aime, look at me." She shifted in her seat so she was facing me directly and struck a pose I imagined she used with clients in tricky situations. Her feet were planted firmly on the floor while she leaned in toward me. "I know it's not your hair, and all of this really stinks. Let's face it. But, honestly, a couple of those wigs look really natural on you. And the main thing is, this is all temporary." She waved her hands in a circle as if encompassing the whole bloody mess.

I took a deep breath and calmed down a little. "Do you think I should go for the real hair one? It's the only one I really like."

"Yes, I do. In the grand scheme of things it won't make much of a difference. And if it makes you feel better right now about this whole rotten deal, then I think it's money well spent," she said.

"Okay, then. Let's get out of here," I said.

I paid the deposit and made arrangements to go back to pick up the wig and potentially have my head shaved when my sister arrived in town. Although I was still undecided about the head-shaving. Everyone just talked about it like it was a given, something that had to be done. I tried to reconcile it in my head, imagining Demi Moore in

G. I. Jane as a total bad ass attacking her own glossy dark hair with a buzzer. There must have been a bad ass inside me somewhere, but I hadn't been in touch with her for a long time. At that point I felt more like a lost child in a carnival fun house, thinking that the fun house wasn't really fun at all.

Jackie and I walked out of the store into the little brick courtyard and paused for a second beside a dripping fountain before we said our good-byes.

"I think you're going to be happy with that decision. It really does look great on you." Jackie nodded, slowly looking into my eyes as if determined for her affirmations to stick.

"Thanks," I said, somewhat skeptically.

"But I've been dying to ask,"—she put her hand on my arm in emphasis—"what happened with the house?"

"Oh, we got it! I'm so excited. We're moving the first weekend in May!" I said, my mood shifting immediately with the mention of it.

Tears sprang up in her eyes, and she pulled me into a hug. "Oh, I'm so happy for you! What a relief!"

It wasn't until that moment that I realized how much she had been worrying. I was suddenly reminded of the first time we met, three years earlier at a new parent function at school. We had just moved from Boston and were still shell-shocked from the transition. Once I met Jackie, we fell into a conversation that was so natural we kept chattering right through a mutual bathroom stop. When we continued our business in side-by-side stalls with Jackie not even breaking stride in the conversation, I knew I had made a friend for life.

And that day, outside of the wig shop, I loved her even more.

CHAPTER 14

All Over Again
Week Three

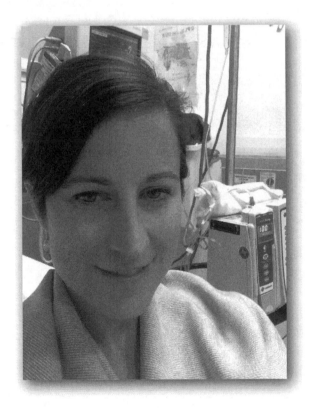

THE NIGHT BEFORE my second round of chemo, my sister Emma called. She was supposed to come out with Lea for the weekend, but Mimi, her new baby, had come down with a bad cold and Emma had a tickle in her own throat. She was at that stage in life where the kids were constantly coming down with something and passing it around the family.

"I'm not sure what to do," she said.

"I don't know, Emma. I know it's hard. It's really up to you."

"Can you check with the doctor to see if it's even okay for me to come when I might expose you to something?" she asked.

"I can check, but she has told me before that it's only advised for me to stay away from people who have an active infection. So, it's a tough call," I said.

I really wanted her to be there, and I was trying to assure her that, but at the same time I was nervous about the way the visit would go. I was worried about wanting to entertain them both and all the little tasks that come along with having people in the house. Where would everyone sleep? Would they find the clean towels and sheets and everything else they might need that I wouldn't be able to get for them? I had always had things set up for guests the same way a hotel would, with everything clean, fresh and laid out properly, but I wasn't capable of putting in that extra effort while I struggled to stay on top of daily household necessities.

I was also heartsick at the thought of missing out while they were hanging out together in my own home, no less. I knew that I would be stuck in a zombie state for the better part of the time they would be there. If one or the other of them were there, it would seem like it was to help, but both together turned into an occasion, something to be celebrated, and I was devastated at the thought of having to miss it. Instead of the prospect of having fun with my sisters for the weekend, I was about to have another round of chemo and dreading it.

We continued to talk it out for several minutes, and I was getting impatient. I didn't think she understood what it was going to be like. I'd been in California for almost three years already, and she still hadn't been able to visit. When she did come, I wanted to have a good visit. I wanted to take her around, to sit and talk with her. The three of us had lately only been able to get together once or twice a year, and those visits centered on helping each other cope with the loss of Mom. At that moment, I had to put that pain aside because I had so much pain of my own—new fears, new panic, and new pain that I couldn't describe to one of the closest people in my life. I tried to explain it to her, and then I finally broke down.

"Emma, you don't understand. I'm going to be sick! Really sick! It's not going to be a nice visit with us hanging around talking and watching movies and drinking wine."

"Sick like the flu? Don't worry about that. I can help. I can take care of you."

"No, it's not sick like the flu. It's worse." I tried to explain it to her, and while I thought through some of the details I felt the panic rising in my chest. I was willingly going to walk into it the next day. I was willingly going to pump my body full of bags and bags of toxicity that would ultimately take my body months and months to completely process, and for the first few days I was fairly certain I would be worthless. "It's much worse," I said, lacking the words or the heart to tell her how bad it could be.

"Just stay home," I finally said. "Stay home and take care of Mimi and come visit when I'm feeling better and I can spend more time with you. Lea will take care of me. It'll be fine. I'll be fine."

After we hung up I threw the phone hard into the soft pillows in frustration. I could not expect Emma to be able to read my mind and anticipate my needs, but I wished she could. I also wished for it to all go away, but I was so deep inside it, I couldn't even let my mind drift to a place where cancer didn't exist.

I wanted her to be there all the time, not just for a visit, and certainly not for this. It was another reminder of how very far away I was from my life. The life I thought I was building in California was not the one that mattered. The deliberation over whether or not she could come help me made my own choices crystal clear. In order to help me, Emma had to leave her sick baby and fly for two full days back and forth across the country. It was too much to ask, but she had been willing to do it. To do what, to hold my hand? To cry with me? It would have been worth it to her, but it was more than I could ask.

The next day I sat in the infusion center again, waiting for my second round of pain. I thought of Susan Sarandon sneaking a puff of a joint in *Stepmother* and that woman in *Beaches* sitting bundled in blankets on an Adirondack chair breathing the fresh air while her body was weakened from cancer and chemotherapy. When did they figure out the dinners and the kid pick-ups and the dog-walking? Was there some mysterious team of people lurking in the shadows attending to their needs?

I was pleased with what I had been able to do the previous week. I went to Fioli with Lauren, took Maverick and the kids up to the park a couple of times, stayed on top of emails and the general coordination of things that I normally did. I was feeling a little bit like myself again. So it was difficult to think of going back to the place I had just climbed out of. The challenge was heightened because I knew exactly how it would feel, unless it was worse. It would be hard, but I knew I could do it. It was like another leg of the race. If I didn't think too hard about it, I would get through.

It reminded me of the days after Mom died when Dad was upset by having all of her clothes in their closet, so he asked my sisters and me to move them to another closet, or take them, or donate them—whatever—as long as he didn't have to face them every time he went into his closet. The process took us three hours as we pulled piles of clothes into one of our old bedrooms. We would stop from time to time when we saw something of Mom's that reminded us of a special occasion.

Emma pulled out a well-worn pair of Lilly Pulitzer pajama pants that conjured countless hours lounging over breakfast in the sunroom, and lost it. "How are we supposed to do this now?" she asked, panic in her wide brown eyes.

"Just don't think about it," I said, mechanically sorting through the piles of shoes. Keep, donate, trash. I had a task to do and I could fall apart later.

"Okay," she said with a quivering breath, and tucked the pajama pants into her own "keep" pile.

I sat on the hospital bed in one of the private rooms in the infusion center because all of the other stations were full. I appreciated the extra space, but I imagined the purpose of the private rooms was for more seriously ill patients or those who were in such a delicate state they required more isolation. I was starting the infusion on my own that day, having assured Scott I would be fine. We agreed that he would come halfway through the process and we would ride home together.

I had made it through the first round pretty well, I told myself. There were some bad days at first, but I had the feeling of having just overcome a bad virus when the adrenaline kicked in, and I was just glad to be in my body again. I was starting to lose a little more hair, but it still looked pretty normal. I believed the women I talked to who had been through this before—that I could do it, that it was manageable. Laura and Catherine's teacher, Brenda, had both boosted my confidence, and if they could do it, so could I. I was still willfully ignoring the warnings from my oncologist that everyone was different. I figured that if everyone was different, maybe I would skate through it. Maybe my experience would be even easier.

I chatted with the nurse while she set up my IV. She brought me down a peg saying, "Yes, hair loss is a symptom. It happens to everyone." She was a different nurse than I'd had before and while she had a prim smile fixed in place, she seemed to almost enjoy being blunt and cutting right to the chase. "See all your hairs on the pillow? Once it starts falling out like that, it won't be long."

"Oh," I said, suddenly seeing at least thirty or forty dark brown strands of hair that had attached themselves to the pillow without my notice. They seemed to make a sound when they fell, like the tinkling of pine needles falling off Charlie Brown's Christmas tree.

"So how are you feeling after round one?" she asked.

"I'm feeling pretty good. The nausea wasn't too bad; the medicines really seemed to do the trick. I had some serious issues going to the bathroom, but once I got that figured out and my fatigue started to go away, I got gradually better each day, and now I'm pretty normal."

"No mouth sores?"

"No, that's been okay. My gums started feeling a little sensitive one day, then I swished with coconut oil and it got better," I said, running my tongue over a slightly tender patch in my mouth.

"How's your appetite?"

"I wouldn't say it's normal, but I've been able to eat. Mostly carbs. Mashed potatoes go down well, and simple things like chicken and rice."

"And your energy?"

"It was very low, especially days three and four, but I've bounced back now. I was able to start walking the dog up our big hill to the park by day six or seven."

"That's good. Remember exercise helps fatigue," she said.

Right. It might have come through my expression, but I didn't say it out loud. The way I felt on days three and four couldn't have been cured by a quick jog, even if I could have made it out the door with my sneakers on. "Thanks. I'll keep that in mind."

"Just remember, there is a cumulative effect, so some of the issues may increase over the next few weeks. Okay? We're all set for now. I'll come check on you in a few minutes and we'll start the Adriamycin push."

"Okay, thanks." I said, letting the words "cumulative effect" bounce around my head for a moment before I pushed them away. As long as it was just a little worse each time, or lasted just a little longer, I'd probably be fine. I dug into my entertainment bag and pulled out my shawl and a magazine.

A few minutes later a knock on the door got my attention, and I looked up to see one of the moms from school, Ellen Atwood. "Hello!" she said. "I hoped I would find you in here!"

"Ellen! I'm so glad you could stop by. Come in!" I waved her into the seat next to the bed, thrilled by her unexpected visit.

"I remember you said you would be in today, and I just finished with my last client next door and wondered if I could catch you." She waved her Stanford ID card and laughed. "Sometimes being on staff has its advantages."

Ellen and I didn't have kids in the same class, so we'd only gotten to know each other sporadically over the previous few years, but every time we spoke, we had much to talk about, so I was glad to have this time to visit with her. Because she was in the healthcare industry herself, she was not put off by the surroundings, and after a brief catch up about my health status, the conversation roamed from books we were reading to fun trips with kids and eventually to school. The middle school issue came up organically, but once it was there, we each had a lot to say on the subject. I filled her in candidly on what had happened with Catherine and that we were planning to move.

"Wow. That's the last thing you want to deal with right now." She sighed, tossing back her hair and running her fingers through it as she looked up toward the ceiling. "You know, I really do worry about the pressure that's put on the kids in this area. Even this middle school application process is much more intense than it needs to be. I don't know how my oldest got into his school. Sometimes it feels like it's just a lottery. It's a lot to have to handle at ten and eleven years old. They're just old enough to be fully aware of the process and have a role in it but much too young to have a healthy perspective. That's if they're even getting a healthy perspective from their parents, which in this environment is not a given," she said, raising her eyebrows.

"It's true. I thought we could come here and not play the game, but it's hard not to get caught up in it. Why wouldn't I want my kids to go to the best school that is available? I want them to have all the advantages I can give them. I guess the problem is that there has been such a huge influx of talent into this area that the infrastructure is having a hard time keeping up," I said.

"The public schools in the good districts are having five or six classes per grade in some cases, and in those districts the housing prices have skyrocketed to a level that is unattainable to all but the very top level of each profession." Ellen shook her head while she spoke and moved out of the way as the nurse brushed by her to start the Adriamycin push.

"I know, Shelley told me the properties start at two million in Menlo Park. These are for places that were built on postage stamp lots as starter homes in the sixties. They probably cost about twenty thousand to build originally. People usually just tear them down and start over."

Ellen shook her head and widened her pale blue eyes. "I guess that makes the Atherton lots start at five or six?"

"Ugh," I responded and we both paused for a moment, "that's just gross." I continued on with my complaints, glad for the distraction of the moment. It was satisfying to speak with someone who understood all the layers of the issue, and Ellen did. "But if you're like us, with a good, quiet girl who could get lost in a huge environment and committed to private schools for that reason, it's hard to find the right place. When we went through the application process at one school, the admissions director explained that the way they choose the incoming class is like making a salad."

Ellen rolled her eyes, "Oh no, they didn't."

"She did. Let me explain. When you're making a good salad you need lots of ingredients. You need some super strong academic children, you need some athletes, you need some musical talent, and you need some diversity, both ethnically and socio-economically. And these are the kids they're choosing for the spots that are available after the siblings, alumni children, staff children, and particularly well-connected children get their crack at it. So take someone like Catherine, a quiet, sweet, smart girl who likes drama and horses, who comes from a nice, well-educated but not super wealthy family, and what does she add to the salad? At best, she's a carrot! There are hundreds of them!" I waved my hands in frustration, and the nurse glanced up at me, happy to let us talk as she continued her work.

"Well, she's not a radish, and this year it was what they needed. That perfect radish." She laughed and put her hand on the bed, "but seriously, I think you guys will be really happy at Woodside, and if you want to try the independent school route again for high school, coming from Woodside Elementary will only be an asset."

"Thanks for talking it out with me, Ellen. You have such a gift at taking just the right tone." I smiled at her, so glad for her company and her advice and finally ready to put the whole issue to rest.

"I aim to please," she said, "but I'd better take off so I can pick up the boys from basketball. Are you okay here?"

"Oh, I'm fine, thank you! Scott should be here any minute. I'm so excited, too, because my sister, Lea, is coming in tonight."

"Oh, that's wonderful! I hope you two get some good restful bonding time. There is nothing better than sisters."

"I agree."

Scott walked in just as Ellen was leaving, and after a few busy moments, we were alone. "Seems like everything is going okay. Do you feel the same?" he asked me.

"So far, so good," I said. "Just talking about school stuff."

"Sorry I missed that one," Scott said, rolling his eyes and getting a giggle from me in response.

I spent the next hour stewing over my conversation with Ellen. People talked about how crazy it was there—it was widely acknowledged—but they always shrugged their shoulders as if they were helpless to do anything about it. They worried endlessly about the effect on their children and attended meetings about the rash of teen suicides, but still maintained these sky-high expectations for themselves and their families. One brilliantly insightful high school student wrote an open letter that was circulated on social media imploring the parents to wake up and see how miserably stressed out she and her peers were. They lived in a constant fear of failure and pressure to succeed on a level that was narrowly defined. For all the parents' good intentions, they seemed to be providing the exact opposite of what their children needed.

I finished up and we picked up the kids on the way home. I caught a glimpse of my face in the side mirror as I looked out the window on the drive up the 280 to San Carlos. With the green ridges and pink evening sky in the backdrop, my face receded in the mirror in a ghostly pallor. I leaned my head back against the seat and closed my eyes. Did it really matter? I could feel myself already starting to drift away again, falling placidly into the dark abyss of nothingness.

By the time Lea arrived that night I was almost asleep, but I heard her come in and went to meet her by the front door.

"Oh, you're still awake! I was thinking you might be too tired." She put her bags down by the front door and hugged me. "How are you feeling?"

"I'm okay," I said. My voice sounded like I was speaking through a tunnel. "Can we sit down?" The walk up the steps to the front door had left me light-headed and winded, but the sight of her soothed me. It had been months since I had seen her, but the way she felt like an extended part of myself never seemed to fade. The years never seemed to catch up to her. Her long, highlighted sandy blonde hair hung straight past her shoulders, and her lithe frame was always draped with the latest casual fashions with a touch of her Southern roots accentuated somehow either by the collection of bracelets on her arm or her distressed leather flats.

"Sure!" she chirped, but I could see the concern hiding in the faint lines around her hazel eyes, the exact color of mine but one shade lighter. Scott picked up her bags and took them to her room, so we could be alone to talk. I don't even remember what we talked about. I was just glad she was there. It was like a part of me that had been missing was complete again.

The plan was for her to stay with me while Scott took the kids for some spring skiing for the weekend. I thought it was the best case scenario. Lea wanted to be there to help, and we could have a lot of time to sit around resting and catching up while Scott and the kids were able to stretch their legs and get away from my being sick for a while. I had heard the second round recovery might be the worst one, and I was grateful that Lea had stepped in to help.

Scott and the kids left early the next morning and I woke to the sounds of Lea busily cleaning up and puttering around the kitchen. I laughed to myself. She never did like to sit still. Her body was in a perpetual state of motion left over from her early years of running track and worrying about her baby sisters. I ambled up the steps and plopped myself down on a stool at the counter. She smiled at me as she finished wiping down the sink. "How are you feeling?"

"Tired. But waking up a bit," I said, rubbing my bleary eyes.

"That's good. Well, what do we need to do today? You mentioned you have to go back in for your booster. What time is that?"

"I have an appointment for 12:30. Then I'm supposed to pick up the wig at 2:30. I could go ahead and shave my head then, too, but I don't know."

She didn't skip a beat. "I'm so glad I can do that with you. Just go ahead and shave it. Didn't you say it would make the wig more comfortable? Then you don't have to worry about it anymore. My friend Elizabeth did that. She said it wasn't that big of a deal, and she was glad she had done it. She actually loved her wigs. Her Facebook picture is still one with the wig on. Look." She grabbed her phone and swiped her finger repeatedly against the screen until she pulled up the photo to show me.

I loved the way she fell into the routine of my life so easily. She had never been to our house, and she was not a nurse, yet there she was, naturally making herself useful and supporting me in an undramatic and casual way, which to me was like butter on bread. Perfect.

We drove to the hospital for my Nupagen shot that was intended to boost my white blood cells, got some green juice at the Juicery, which I was pleased to be able to get down, and made our way back to the wig store in San Carlos. By that time I had thought about it long enough. I was ready to take the plunge and shave my head. The fact that I was sick of my *House of Cards* hairdo, which my dad said made me look like a news anchor, helped a little.

I had warned Lea that the stylists at the place were rude, so she brought her extra sweet Southern charm on and warmed them up. I sat in the chair, and the stylist started buzzing.

"Oh, do you want me to take a couple of pictures?" Lea stood in front of me leaning against the counter with her back toward the mirror I was looking into, her hand reaching for her phone.

The stylist paused, having just started in the back.

"Um, sure." I had been wincing a bit at the noise and the mental pain of the business, so I broke into a tentative smile.

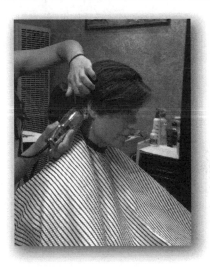

Click. Documented. The stylist continued shaving my head in swift motions from back to front in a way that reminded me of watching the gardener mow our lawn in Massachusetts. Straight lines, he never missed a blade; he even crisscrossed the front lawn to leave a pretty pattern. There was nothing pretty about what was left on my head. The bump from an injury I'd had as a child was in high relief, and the black stubble that was left behind stood out harshly against my paper white scalp.

I rubbed my hand over it a couple of times.

"Can I feel it?" Lea asked eagerly, making me laugh a little.

I nodded and she ran her hand over the top of my head. I glanced up at her, wrinkling my nose. "It's cool!" she assured me, "it's sort of velvety, right?"

"Maybe." I hesitated. "Let's do the wig now."

We got the wig fitted just right, and I never showed my shaved head in public again.

Lea drove my car from the San Carlos town center up the side of the hills to our house, relying on my navigation to guide her through the maze of one-way streets that wound up the side of Devonshire Canyon. Scott and I had the habit of parking in the driveway that barely held both of our cars because I had let the kids convert the garage into a giant Legoland in lieu of a playroom. From the front, the house looked like it was a little one-room cabin, but if you walked around the corner down the hill, three stories rose out of the earth in a great expanse of stucco. Lea stopped the car and handed me the keys, and I fumbled with the old lock on the heavily carved wooden front door.

"It's a cute neighborhood," she said, looking around at the other houses on the street. "I can see the attraction." Her eyes fixed on the driveway across the street, carved into the side of the hill and sloping steeply up toward a garage and another flight of stairs leading up to the front door. "Have you met any of your neighbors?"

I followed her gaze and looked at the big stucco house. "Well, in that house there are a bunch of kids who work at GoPro. They're all in their twenties and they're pretty funny. They invited Scott to a party once when I was gone, and he had a couple of beers and had to leave when they started playing drinking games. He said they were way out of his league. They're always strapping surfboards and mountain bikes on their trucks in the afternoons and heading out somewhere. See those vans?"

I pointed to two old sketchy-looking vans that were parked on the street a little further down the block. She nodded and I went on. "Those belong to a couple of their friends. They're living in them. They thought they were beating the housing game and being clever, but the guys in the house get annoyed when they come in to use the shower. I hear all the scoop because one of their girlfriends babysits for us."

She laughed. "It's like something out of a movie."

I agreed. "Silicon Valley. It's entertaining just living here."

I opened the door and Maverick greeted us with a low woof and a thumping of his tail on the floor. I sank into the couch, and Lea flipped on the TV.

"Want to watch a movie?"

"Sure, why don't you pick something," I said, looking down at my phone. "I just have to text the pot delivery guy to see if he can bring over those edibles he said he was getting in."

"What?" Lea asked, turning her face towards me with the exaggerated affectation of a scandalized expression. "So, really? I get to meet him? What's he like?" She peppered me with excited questions.

I giggled, thinking back to when I met Mike a couple of weeks before. After I got what I jokingly referred to as my pot card, I searched medical marijuana dispensaries on Google and found a map of Silicon Valley dotted with little green leaves indicating delivery services. The main dispensaries were in San Francisco and San Jose, but there were individual distributors in several locations in between. I looked at the different profiles and chose one from nearby Redwood City. My hand shook with nerves as I dialed the number listed, but Mike answered the phone and immediately put me at ease once he determined my situation. "I have had a lot of clients going through that too," he said, "I can bring over some samples that might help you out."

I asked him to come by the house when Scott was home, and we made sure the kids were otherwise occupied in their rooms. Mike strolled into our living room wearing shorts and a polo shirt and spread out a briefcase full of weed on our coffee table. He helped me chose a few different kinds to try that he said were "pretty mellow" and left me with a handful of plastic pouches labeled with names like Kush and U2, so that I could keep track of what I liked or didn't like. "We're running a special where you get a free joint with a purchase of thirty five dollars or more," he told me and gave me a perfectly rolled fat little joint encased in a tube.

Over the next couple of weeks I tried some of the different kinds, but I still wasn't sure what it was doing for me. I supposed that it might be fun to zone out a little bit, but I didn't really want to escape from my life. I wanted to hold onto it. I hadn't put a dent in what I had purchased from Mike yet, but I had done some research that suggested that the main benefit from Cannabis was the Cannabidiol content or CBD. The CBDs could be separated from THC, which was the property that caused a high. I had read that CBD chews could be helpful with sleep and relaxation without causing any psychotropic side effects so I called Mike back and he let me know he was getting some in this week. I thought I should give it a try.

"Actually, he's pretty cute," I responded to Lea. "Tall, fit, clean cut, a lot younger than I thought he'd be."

Twenty minutes later Lea jumped up to answer the door and escorted Mike, with his suitcase full of pot, into our kitchen. We all sat around the table while he showed me the latest in edibles he'd just gotten. Mike and I launched into a conversation discussing the potential benefits of each kind and the different health conditions they might be able to treat. Lea looked back and forth between us while she seemed to be perpetually stifling a giggle.

I chose a handful of toffee-like candies that Mike warned me to "only take a slice of," and we said goodbye. Lea closed the door behind him and turned to me, her eyes dancing with mischief.

"Well, that was something new," she said. "He was cute. And he didn't look like a stoner at all. Are you going to have some now?"

"I'll probably wait until I want to go to sleep. Why? Do you want some?" I teased her.

"Not for me. It might make me paranoid," she said, waving her hands in protest. "I do think it's about time for a glass of wine, though, after all that!"

I nodded, already drained from the activity. "Help yourself," I said, snuggling deep into the couch and putting my head down on the pillow. That was the last thing I remembered about that day.

CHAPTER 15

—— ✣ ——

Second Round Knockdown

SATURDAY AND SUNDAY passed in a haze. I would wake for short bits of time and struggle out of my bed to talk to Lea and get a bite of food. I was weighed down from the pain and the head fog that seemed more pronounced from the second round. I had experienced head rushing on the first round, but it had been much more subtle, so much that I didn't bother to include it when describing my symptoms to the medical team. Before it had felt like I was on a strong round of antibiotics, or had had too much coffee, or was sleep deprived, but the second bout was much more intense. It felt like my ears were stopped up with water, and there was a constant noise in my head. When I stood up it would increase, then subside slightly when I sat down. The only thing that would make it go away entirely was sleep.

Lea kept herself busy helping out and catching up on her reading. She walked Maverick up to the park for me, enjoying the exercise and telling me about the neighbors she met. She said she was careful to avoid the huge Bernese Mountain puppy that I had warned her Maverick didn't like because the puppy would chase him and try to jump on Maverick's back. His name was Bruce. Even the sound of his name made Maverick curl up his lip in a menacing growl. Lea seemed to think the conflict added an exciting element to the task, her job to save Maverick from the battle of the beasts.

Jackie stopped by, and we all sat out on the deck in the lounge chairs under the eucalyptus trees for a visit. We talked for a few minutes and I started to fade. Two of my favorite people, my sister and Jackie, were finally meeting, but my heart sank as my energy weakened and eventually I lay down on the couch and drifted off while they chatted in the kitchen. I wasn't trying to listen in, but pieces of their conversation reached me before I slept.

"I'm glad to see her. I had to make sure she was doing okay. How does she seem to you?" Jackie asked.

"She's okay. I can tell it's pretty tough on her. She hates being vulnerable," Lea said.

"I know, I can tell it's hard for her to ask for help. We've been concerned that she might not ask for something that she needs."

"Oh really? I think she'd speak up if there was something you could do. I'm sure she just wants to cave up and sleep."

"I don't know. I'm not really available during the week, but Lauren has said she's been trying to reach out, and Aime hasn't been that responsive. She said she's been trying to get her out for walks, but she's only gotten her to do things once or twice. But, I get it. When I'm feeling bad, I just want to stay home, too," Jackie said.

"I don't think she really needs someone to take her on a walk. She'll get out if she wants to." Lea said protectively.

"Well, I told Lauren there was a big difference between Aime wanting to go to Fioli, where all the ladies go to walk the gardens and lunch, and just getting out in the neighborhood. One of my colleagues had mentioned that his wife had gotten a little homebound during her treatment, and he liked it when her friends would come get her out for some fresh air, but Lauren keeps wanting to take her to fancy places that require a lot of energy and dressing up and all."

"That's really sweet that she's concerned," Lea responded. "But it's not like that. Aime's fine. I guarantee you the main thing she wants right now is just to be left alone. Check in every now and then, but give her a lot of space. That's always how she is when anything bad happens. She seems to be getting out on her good days. I'm really glad that she has you girls, though. It really makes me feel better knowing you'll be looking out for her."

"We love her and we'd do anything to help. I only wish we could do more."

Eventually Jackie said goodbye and the rest of the night fell into oblivion.

On Sunday I mentioned I could use another hat, and Lea went out immediately looking for one. She came back an hour later with a blue terrycloth turban tucked over her long blonde highlighted hair. I giggled immediately while she looked at me and deadpanned, "What?" Then she laughed and tossed it off her head, explaining the only place she could find a hat was the wig shop, and it was the best they had.

I slept for hours that day and Lea came into my room periodically to offer food or just sit next to me on the bed and watch TV for a while. The head rushing had become intense whenever I stood. Once after going to the bathroom, when I stood up to take the five steps back to my bed, a tugging sensation pulled at the side of my cheek as if a string were attached to the corner of my mouth and someone was trying to sew it to my ear.

The aches and pains flared up in my joints and bones, particularly in my sternum, adding to the tenderness in my chest from the surgery. It was so difficult to isolate the symptoms and pain to determine what was caused by the chemotherapy versus the booster shot versus the initial surgery because everything felt wrong.

On her way to the airport Monday, Lea dropped me off for an ultrasound. I was starting to feel better, expecting to feel better, but I was still very weak. I cried as she left, thinking the visit was too short, that I had wasted so much of it sleeping, wishing, oh, wishing that she could be closer, that I could have her with me through this. It was such a harsh blow that I had to do this without her or my mom or anyone who had ever really known how to take care of me. I think her visit had propped up my energy by Monday, but watching her leave I felt it start to vanish with her, and then I was left alone.

Fatigue is such a vague word. When I think of fatigue, I imagine a feeling of depletion as if I had stayed out in the sun too long or had a bad sleep the previous night. The way I felt was as if I lay at the bottom of a deep chasm and could not even lift my face toward the light at the top of it. I didn't really feel *anything*. It was the absence of feeling that was so difficult. I understood what it felt like to die. You just slip away. I saw that decision in front of me, but I never had to make the choice. Eventually, inch by inch I was able to lift my gaze and see that yes, there was a beautiful life up there, and someday I could reach it again, even though the path was still unclear.

Scott and the kids came home that afternoon full of energy and excitement from their skiing adventure. Scott looked at my hat as he dropped a bag on the floor.

"Oh, you did it," he said. I looked at him blankly and then remembered my shaved head and nodded. The kids were curious about my head for about a second until they agreed it was fine if I had a hat on. They moved immediately on to telling me stories about their adventures skiing.

"Catherine ate too many hot dogs and threw up all over the room. Daddy thought it might have been the altitude," Wesley said.

"We learned how to play pool but had to quit when Wesley hit me with the pool stick," Catherine said.

Scott laughed and pulled out his phone, showing me the pictures. Smiling faces and arms spread in front of mountains, in villages with ice cream cones, in front of a pot of fondue.

I tried to focus and nod and ask questions in the appropriate places, but even that ruse only lasted a few moments before I had to go back to bed. The rushing in my head had gotten stronger, and I was having a hard time concentrating on the quick banter.

I held on tightly to the railing down the stairs to the bedroom and felt like I was walking on a balloon. I reached the bathroom and my reflection in the mirror caught my attention. I stared at this person in the glass and searched for myself, but I couldn't find me. My eyes looked dead tired, even vacant. All the life had been sucked out of them, all of the sparkle, the vibrancy, the vitality. It was all gone. I saw flat, lifeless eyes sunken into a pallid face staring back at me without expression, without even fear or horror at what they saw.

I shuffled a few more steps and buried myself in my bed. My instincts had always been to bring the kids into the bed when they were sick or had a nightmare. Somehow it seemed to have almost magical powers of healing. Mama and Daddy's bed. At that moment it felt like the last place on earth that I could exist. I hoped and prayed that the magic would work for me.

In the early evening, a nurse called with the ultrasound results and told me that all of my lymph nodes appeared normal.

"Oh, thanks," I said quietly into the phone.

"It's good news. I just thought you would want to know."

"Okay," I said and hung up. I was so deep into my fog that the news hadn't even really registered with me. I stared out the window, watching the black squirrel run up and down the tree trunk, then stretch out and rest next to a knot on the limb.

The light changed from evening to night while I alternated between staring vacantly out the window and toward the cavernous bathroom and closet.

Scott and I had joked about the way the room had been built—the progression of the construction was clearly piece by piece. What had started as a closet turned into a vanity and little bathroom, then the closet was pushed further into the side of the hill when more space was created for a large Jacuzzi complete with royal blue tile and mirrored walls, which must have been an eighties addition, and a walk-in closet that Scott had to duck his head to get into. Each feature burrowed into the side of the canyon like the nest of a rodent. I think at that moment I appreciated the cold, dark sunken retreat in an animal instinct to curl up and die.

I passed two more days that way before I finally to started to question what was going on. I came back into myself enough to realize how far gone I had been. My survival instinct suddenly kicked in, and I was spoiling for a fight. I started searching the message boards about symptoms for my particular brand of chemo, at the same time realizing what the results of the ultrasound might mean. I put the pieces together in such a way that I saw for the first time that I was undergoing one of the most intensive forms of chemotherapy available, and as far as anyone knew for certain, the cancer was already gone.

I thought of Laura, the funny nanny who convinced me that I could just stay high through the whole thing, then I thought of Catherine's teacher who had said it would be okay. It'll be hard, she said, but it's mostly just feeling sick and tired. But this was different. This was awful. This was indescribable. This was killing me cell by cell. If either of them had felt close to how I felt right at that moment, they would never have described it so cheerfully. I didn't want any more pep talks. It was quite apparent to me that everyone's experience was in fact different, and mine particularly sucked.

I pulled my stash of pot out of the bedside dresser drawer and loaded up the vaporizer with a fresh bowl. I inhaled slowly and deeply letting the herb percolate in the steam like the man at the smoke shop had instructed me to do and waited for the pain to go away. It didn't. I threw the pipe on the bed in disgust. It did nothing for me. I was so loaded up with other drugs that I couldn't even feel it. As much as it sounded like fun, I wasn't going to smoke my way through this one. I walked into the bathroom and picked up my bottle of Ativan. The only relief I could get was by shutting down my brain. I looked at the clock on my phone. 12:32 p.m. Three hours until the kids would be home. Eight hours until I could slip into oblivion. I would have to wait. The hours crawled by until bedtime.

I don't know if it's my personality or how I was raised or both, but as long as I can remember I have been uncomfortable making a big deal out of pain. When Wesley was born, I felt the contractions start and called Lea, wanting to talk through it with her before I decided it was really time.

I held my breath for an extra few seconds on the phone and she said, "Yes, that's definitely it. The real thing." She knew me so well and knew that the telling signal would be just that sharp intake of breath.

My mom had been with me. I had waited to tell her until I was sure. We left Catherine with the sitter and I called Scott at work, asking him to meet me at the hospital while Mom drove me over the bridge from Charlestown to Mass General. We all got to triage at the same time and the nurse checking in sat behind the counter, gave me a once over, and asked me to wait. After I had been waiting about fifteen minutes another woman came into triage being pushed by her husband in a wheelchair and making all kinds of noise. The crew I thought I was waiting for bustled around her and got her into an exam room.

Mom and I glanced at each other and she pointedly looked at the woman behind the admitting desk.

"I guess I have to scream and cry to get a room," I said, shaking my head.

Scott stood up and paced restlessly in front of our chairs, and we waited for another half an hour. When I was finally brought into a room and examined the nurse popped her head up over the sheet draped across my thighs and said, "Did you want an epidural?"

"Yes, I had planned on it. It's getting really uncomfortable now," I said.

"I'm going to get the anesthesiologist in right away. You're very close. He'll tell us if there is time."

They wheeled me in the triage bed down to the delivery room, administering the epidural on the way, and Wesley was born twenty minutes later. Mom came in the room hours later and told me the other woman had just had her baby. She winked at me. I sniffed, and then we shared a giggle.

I'll admit, having a second child can be far less dramatic than the first, but Wesley was born weighing over nine pounds and his strong kick cracked one of my ribs on the way out. He had a bruise for a month on his little foot to prove it. I'm just not a screamer. I never have been. But chemotherapy had broken me. I was finally ready to scream.

CHAPTER 16

❧

Fighting Back

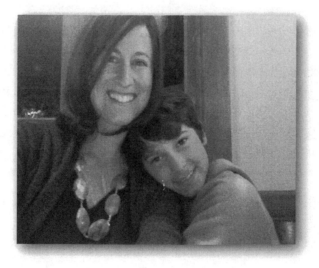

I CALLED TRIAGE. I cried on the phone to the nurse. Finally Dr. S called me.

"I hear you're having a hard time," she said.

"The chemo is going to kill me. It's too much. I can't do two more rounds. I won't make it. I'm not even sure I need this. Why am I on the heaviest possible chemo there is? How did this happen? You said Gold Standard, not industrial strength. Didn't I explain to you that I can't even drink coffee without getting jittery?" I was barely keeping my rising voice under control.

"Well, we discussed this based on your pathology from the surgery. It's the standard, and there is no question that your particular pathology combined with your age receives the best long-term results with this chemotherapy regime," Dr. S said.

"I know there are other types of chemo. Why am I doing the hardest one when I don't even know for sure that there is cancer left in my body?"

"Yes, there are other options, but we chose this one for you based on the research that we have."

"I don't remember ever having the choice. This was presented to me as the only option," I said, lowering my voice slightly.

"Well, there is always a choice. You are in the driver's seat here and there are options. I can recommend what I think is best for you based on a long-term strategy, but I can't make you do it. Remember, this is not just for now, but we are trying to give you the best chance to live the longest life possible. This is a long-term strategy, a decades-long strategy."

"But what good is this strategy if I don't make it past the treatment? Everyone keeps talking about the cumulative effect. *I won't make it* two more rounds." The constant rushing in my head that increased when I bent over, the slight tugging sensation in my right cheek, the numbness in my left arm—any of these things could trigger my death. Heart attack, stroke, blood clot. The endless litany of peril circled through my head.

"Let's see how you come out of it in the next few days, and when I see you next Thursday we'll decide how to move forward. Aime, you're going to be okay. We're going to get through this. You should know that this is easily one of the hardest things that you will ever have to do. It's toxic shit. There is a reason why we don't give it to everyone. But I think you should do it, and I think you can."

I had asked Shelley to bring the kids home from school that day. I had been camped out on the couch and heard their footsteps run toward the front door. I opened the door to greet them and waved at Shelley. She blew me a kiss and got back into the car, somehow knowing I wasn't up for a chat.

We got through the afternoon, and I pulled out a prepared dinner for the kids, picking at a few bites myself. I had my favored big fluffy wool beanie hat pulled over my head instead of my wig, and Wesley patted it as he sat down.

"Softie," he grinned.

"Do you mind if I don't wear a wig?" I asked him, as always concerned about the impact of my changing appearance on him.

"It's fine," he said raising his thin shoulders up and down in a shrug. "I don't want to see your head, though. Without hair."

"Okay, yeah. I don't really blame you." I agreed, not really thinking he needed to see it.

"You know, it's funny, though." He gave me another huge grin and pointed his finger in the air waiting to make sure I was paying attention.

"What's that?"

"I don't have my front teeth, and you don't have your hair." He laughed triumphantly, assured that he had made a fine point. He opened his mouth in an exaggerated smile to give me the best view of the gummy space where his two baby teeth had recently been. The new teeth were starting to poke through, huge and a little crooked.

"You're right!" I laughed. I ruffled his hair, relishing his thick and soft dark brown locks.

Catherine had been watching the exchange uninterested, then piped in, "And I'll bet they'll be growing back about the same time." She gave me a sweet smile and nudged Wesley under the table.

Scott texted to let me know he would be a little late and to see if there was any takeout I might want. The pile-up at work was catching up with him, and he had to grab the extra hours when he could. But by Wesley's eight o'clock bedtime I was completely drained again. I lay down on my bed after dinner and only got up to ask him to take his shower. By bedtime it took all my strength to shuffle down the hallway and tuck him into bed.

"Baby song," he reminded me as if I would ever forget.

"There is a young cowboy who lives on the range," I started in with the first few notes of Sweet Baby James by James Taylor, a song

I had sung thousands of times. Wesley settled right down and buried himself into the covers.

"Night, night, Mama."

"Night, night, Wesley. I love you."

"So do I." He smiled and turned to face the wall, cuddling his little Lamby next to his face and closing his eyes.

I pulled his door closed and shuffled back down the carpeted hallway, peeking in on Catherine as I passed her door.

"Hey sweetie, I need to lie down for a little bit. Dad will be home soon. Can you keep an eye on the time for me in case I fall asleep before your bedtime?

She looked up from her place sprawled on her polka dotted bedspread, strategically positioned between an array of pillows and stuffed animals. "Okay. I'll come tell you when it's time for me to go to bed."

"Thanks, sweetheart. I love you."

"I know." She smiled and looked back down at her homework.

I pulled the covers over my head and sank into my bed again, muffling my sobs with the pillow so Catherine couldn't hear. I was doing the best I could and hoped, please dear God, that it was enough and that everyone would get through this okay.

On days five and six I went through the motions numbly, slowly starting to regain my strength. I was left with a bone-tired fatigue. Simple things would leave me breathless such as walking up the stairs or taking a shower. I wasn't even close to carrying out a normal day. I had a constant fluid drip from my nose, and the whites of my drooping eyes had turned yellow and were rimmed with red. My vision was blurred, I had a constant tightness in my chest, heart palpitations, numbness in my fingertips that sometimes stretched up my arm, and a pain at the base of my skull that reached around to my right ear. I had lost five more pounds, but my ankles were puffy in a way that my acupuncturist had told me indicated kidney strain. I wrote out a list of symptoms on my phone, because the head fog was starting to become a problem.

By Thursday morning, one full week after round two, I woke with slightly better energy and attempted to regain some control of my life. I mentally ran over the mounting list of tasks. We had planned to go to Carmel for Easter and were scheduled to leave the next day, and of course I needed to prepare for our move back to Woodside. As much as I enjoyed San Carlos, I wished we had never left Woodside. I remembered the damp, moldy house buried in the redwoods we rented for an astronomical price for the first two years and knew we had to get out of that place, but we weren't able to find another house there and landed in San Carlos. I thought it would be a good move to a sunnier place—with all the open air from the deck, wide open sky, and views over the canyon—but the longer drive back and forth between school and San Carlos had already put an extra strain on us even before I had gotten sick.

I went out to the deck and sank into my favorite chair, breathing in the eucalyptus scent as if it would clear my head and prepare me to face the tasks ahead. If I was starting to feel better that day, I figured I had one week to get everything squared away for the move, minus the next morning, in which I would prepare for Carmel, and the weekend spent in Carmel.

I wasn't sure how we would get it done, but I knew we would. We had to. My brain was working overtime trying to figure out the logistics of the move. I'd done it twice in the last three years. What was once more? Getting Catherine settled into a great school district where she had a friend was the top priority, and we were all happy about moving back to Woodside. Maverick would enjoy the space the most. I could hire out the packing, and Shelley had offered the help of her contractors with getting all the utilities squared away. We could do this. We would. Somehow.

The first few notes of the Beatles playing *Here Comes the Sun* filled the air, and I glanced at my phone.

"Hi, Fronda." I picked up immediately, a habit left over from my mother's sick days. An unexpected call from Nashville always had me on edge for a split second.

"Aime? How are you doing?" My sister-in-law's Texas drawl filled the line.

"Doing well. I've pulled through the second round. Now I just have to do it two more times, then moving on to the lighter stuff, so they say."

"Well, that's good. Um, I do have some news of my own to share." My heart sank. I didn't want to hear it.

"It turns out that I have breast cancer too." What? I leaned forward in my chair, clutching my stomach and trying to get air back into my lungs. This couldn't be happening. Not to both of us. Not at the same time. I pulled myself together, and we talked about the details. We were both shocked. I tried to be encouraging, telling her it wasn't that bad, but we both knew I was lying.

"It's funny, in a terrible sort of way," she said. "I was thinking of Marion's robe today and sort of wishing I still had it." I bristled for a moment before I tucked the ugly feeling away.

"Oh. I wear it all the time. I love having it. I'm so grateful that you sent it to me," I said.

"I know. When I sent it I was thinking it might be something we could pass around if we ever needed to. You know, sort of like the sisterhood of the traveling pants or something," she said, and I let out an uneasy laugh, thinking *That's MY robe! I need it!*

The build-up of problems and worries was mounting to a level I could no longer handle. There was nothing I could do for Fronda. If this had only happened to her the following year, or any other time, or never! If it were just a few months later, I would have been able to help her, to offer her advice and support, and to give her all the tips and tricks that I had learned, but I didn't have anything to give her then.

That hopeless, helpless feeling snaked back into my brain of being so far away from my family. I wanted to be there. I wanted us to be able to share the resources of the family, to be able to lean on each other, but I had to shut it down because it wasn't possible. Fronda would be okay. She had all of my family with her in Nashville as well as her own mother, sisters, and healthy grandmother and a slew of lifelong friends—facts that I had to check myself to not feel bitter about.

I only had myself, Scott, and a handful of new friends. So I sent Fronda the love, prayers, and encouragement that I could, and then I had to let it go.

Then, as if often does, a new day brought a fresh approach, and Friday morning was quite productive. I had managed to get the kids to pack themselves for the weekend the night before and threw some of my own things into a bag. I was becoming pretty adept at the art of out-sourcing. There might not be an easier place to manage a family of four plus animals from a smartphone than in Silicon Valley. I scheduled Maverick's boarding stays, including chauffer service (which was a nice way to call throwing a bunch of dogs in the back of a van and charging twenty dollars per head); Pluto's stay at the cat hotel during the move; packers; movers; and utilities—all from the comfort of my deck chair.

Theresa, our house cleaner, had graciously agreed to help get me organized. It was good fortune that she had a girl slightly younger than Catherine and a boy younger than Wesley. She and her husband, Daniel, were also near Scott's and my sizes, so I was able to give her bags and bags of clothes and toys and things that we no longer need-ed. I think she was doing me a favor more than she wanted the stuff, but it lightened our load significantly, and I was starting to feel opti-mistic about the whole process. We could do this.

It was Good Friday, so the kids had an early release from school after a family chapel. I was feeling pretty strong after all I'd been able to accomplish that morning, so I made a point to be there in time for chapel. Wesley and Catherine both waved to me as they went in, and from their faces I knew my effort to be there had made a difference to them. It was hot that day, and the sun had been bearing down on us while we waited in the courtyard to enter the chapel behind the students. The air was stuffy inside too, and despite the dark wood paneling, the sun filtering through the glass panels of the atrium seemed to work like heat lamps, causing an array of hot spots that dotted the pews. I sat with Jackie and Chris, and as we chatted about meeting up in Carmel my skin started to grow damp and clammy.

"It's so hot today." I said, fanning myself with a program.

Jackie nodded. "It'll be nice in Carmel. Warm during the day, but cool at night. Boots and sweaters for the beach."

As we rose and sat several times through the progression, I leaned heavily against the pew in front of me and looked at Jackie.

Her eyes widened when she saw my face, and she whispered, "Honey, do you need to sit down?"

I nodded and sat for the rest of the song. When she sat next to me again, she asked me what was wrong.

"I think it's just the heat." I shook my head and ran a hand over my forehead, starting to see little black spots at the edge of my vision.

"Have you eaten anything today?" I shook my head again, and she touched my forehead, "Go get something to eat and sit in the air conditioning for a little bit. I'll cover for you here."

As soon as she offered the solution, I knew I had to get out of there. She and Chris stepped out of the way, and I hurried out to my car. I found a bottle of water on the back seat and dug out a Power Bar from my purse. I forced myself to take a few sips and bites and blew the air conditioning at top speed on my face for the remainder of chapel. Just as families started streaming out the door, I was starting to breathe normally again.

I walked back toward the courtyard to pick up the kids and fought back tears. It was all of the simple things that I was missing. Just being able to watch my children sing in chapel and run happily out of school before a break. Cancer was taking all of this away from me, but these were the things that I wanted to hold onto.

Scott met us at home after a couple of hours, and we all piled into the car for the trip. I made it through the two-hour ride by sucking on ginger chews to tamp down my nausea, and I collapsed on the hotel bed while Scott took the kids for a walk around town when we arrived. I could tell Scott was nervous about how I was feeling. Chris had told him about my near pass out in the chapel that morning, but I deflected his pointed questions and assured him I was fine. I would be fine. I wanted to be there.

Carmel-by-the-Sea is a special place for us. Between walks through the cobblestone streets, window shopping at the sweet boutiques and art galleries, playing in the oaks by the beach and some big healthy meals, we all started to feel right by Saturday afternoon. We had plans to meet Jackie and Shelley with their families down at the beach for a cookout. Jackie and Chris had streamlined the beach bonfire process over the years of their homeownership in Carmel, and we were glad to benefit from their expertise.

We met up with Chris at the top of the winding staircase that cut through the cliff down to the sand below. The beach stretched out before us, its white sand in sparkling contrast to the dark blue waters and brighter blue sky. A few puffy clouds dotted the skyline as if their only purpose was to add some artistic flair to the canvas.

Chris had pulled his car up to the sidewalk, popped the trunk, and started unloading a huge supply of firewood, chairs, blankets, coolers, and bags and bags of goodies. I had sent the kids ahead with our own armloads of gear and set down the blanket I was toting to return Chris's big bear hug.

"How're ya doing, girl? I'm so glad to see you!" he said with his deep Southern drawl as he pulled away and gave me a winning smile. "Here, give me a hand with this stuff, Scott, won't you? And Aime, Jackie's already down at the beach. You let us boys take care of the heavy lifting."

I gladly agreed and made my way down the steep stone steps that hugged the side of the bluff. When I got to the bottom of the staircase, Catherine waved at me from farther down the beach and pointed around to the left, where I caught sight of Jackie setting up a folding table and chairs.

My boots sank into the deep sand, and I shed my jacket from the heat of the effort. The sun peeked in and out of the clouds, giving just the right amount of late afternoon warmth and light. Jackie lifted her head as she spread out a tablecloth and caught sight of me.

"You made it!" She bounced a couple of steps through the sand to give me a hug.

"I'm so glad we're doing this. Thank you so much!" I returned her embrace.

"The kids are off," she laughed, pointing at James, Wesley, and Catherine, already chasing the surf and gathering clumps of seaweed.

"What can I do to help?" I asked her, looking around at the tidy site she had arranged.

"I think we're in good shape. Help me get into this bottle of wine?"

The thought of alcohol turned my stomach, and I shook my head. "I'd better stick with water."

"Well, let's sit then. Shelley and family are on their way, and we can start pulling some food together then. So for now it's just us." We sat and talked, laughing at the kids' antics and watching the guys prepare for the fire. Shelley, her husband Jim, and their daughter Abby arrived after a few minutes, and we passed the evening sitting around the fire, roasting hot dogs for dinner and s'mores for dessert as the sky changed slowly from gray to pink to a deep night blue.

I sat back for a moment and looked at my friends and family gathered together around the fire. As pairs huddled close together against the incoming chilly air, I noticed that my perspective started to shift. Catherine and Abby sat bundled under a big blanket playing some kind of girly game while Wesley and James took turns throwing seaweed poppers into the fire. The guys all talked and laughed loudly, taking turns making their way to the cooler for beer. Shelley, Jackie, and I passed away the hours as if they were mere seconds, musing on life, love, children, and happy things. I was being shown in Technicolor what mattered in my life, and the key was to let the other stuff fall away so that on the other side of the struggle my life would be streamlined like I hoped our little cottage would be. I could let go of anything that I didn't love or that didn't make me happy. Isn't that what the experts say about decluttering the home? It was like a hoarders intervention for my life, and I could see myself letting go. The frantic pace of keeping up and all the things I thought I needed but that really only cluttered my life melted away in the firelight.

CHAPTER 17

Moving On

Week Five

I CAN'T BELIEVE I'm here again, I thought, not quite sure how I had done it—how I had ordered the Uber, gotten into the car, and walked into the hospital. Every fiber in my being screamed at me that the chemo was too much, the levels too high. Tears brimmed in my eyes threatening to spill as I pulled out my phone. I had already had my port accessed and blood test done, and I was waiting to be called in to see Dr. S. I grabbed a tissue from the conveniently placed box on the side table. A lot of tears were shed in that place.

I typed out a quick blast on CareZone to friends and family. "I'm at Stanford for round three. I'll be meeting with the surgeon and oncologist, and I'm hoping that I'll have a dosage adjustment due to my weight loss and my reaction last time—the extreme fatigue was a little worrisome all around. Could you all please say a prayer for me today and for the health care team, that we all work together to make the right call. Love to you all!"

I sat there alone and reached out to my people near and far, asking them in my own way for support. Immediately my phone started lighting up with the notifications of responses on CareZone.

"Thinking and praying!" from Lea.

"I just prayed and will continue. God is good and loves you. We all do too. Dad"

"I am praying! Good luck! I love you!" from Emma.

A nurse called my name and introduced herself. "How are you doing today?"

"Okay," I said, wondering why they always ask that. They knew why I was there; I was not really that great.

She punched the big silver plate that opened the automatic door and shuffled me around the corner. "First let's get your height and weight."

I stepped on the scale, it was one of those huge square scales with railings that reminded me of the veterinary scale that weighed our Great Dane when I was a kid that I think was used for livestock.

"56.1kg. Now turn around and let me get your height, please." I tried to mentally calculate the kilograms to pounds and gave up.

"Could you give me the conversion, please?"

"Yep, just a minute. Okay. 5'5, 127 pounds."

"5'5? I've never been 5'5. There must be a mistake. Could you please measure again?"

"Okay," she said and measured carefully. "Yep. 5'5."

Anger welled up and I tried to keep it in check as I ranted inside. 5'5! I've never been 5'5. What, am I shrinking too? Fine. Just add that to the list of symptoms. I've always been 5'6ish, and once I even measured 5'7. This has to be a mistake. I fumed as I followed the nurse to the room.

"We'll be in here," she said, gesturing. "Now let's get your vitals. Do you have an arm you prefer?" I held out my right arm, and she wrapped it with the stiff Velcro blood pressure monitor.

"Now your other hand." She clamped the oxygen monitor on my left index finger. "And your temperature." She pulled the thermometer out and I opened my mouth automatically to let her place it under my tongue. We both watched the machine in silence as the numbers in each dial rose until the loud beep signaled the test's completion. Dismayed, I let her unstrap my arm and take the tools away in silence. I was watching my leverage for a lower dosage slip away from me. I had inexplicably gained a couple of pounds back the previous week, probably due to that beautiful Easter weekend in Carmel, and seemingly lost an inch, so the height/weight factor was not in my favor.

We mechanically went through my ever-lengthening list of medications to make sure it was all current, and I was reminded of my first visit when I was asked to list my medications on a form, and I had nothing to write.

"Okay. Dr. S will be in shortly. Just undress from the waist up and leave the gown open in the front."

I passed the time playing solitaire on my phone while I waited a solid half an hour on the table. I had thought I could do all of this alone. I thought that I could minimize the impact on the family by dividing our resources and not wasting them on "non-essentials" like company for a doctor's appointment, but it was starting to get a little tough. I still wasn't ready to admit it, though, and didn't know what I could do about it anyway. Finally the RN came in with a gentle smile and introduced herself. She was new, and she seemed nice, but she made the mistake of asking, "So how are you doing today?"

I unleashed a barrage of complaints, consulting the list on my phone to make sure I had them all straight. I talked in great detail about each symptom, describing the feelings carefully. It felt as if it were my job to make her understand, to make her feel some part of what I was feeling. Fatigue was inadequate as a word. I had been so "tired" for lack of a better word that it was an effort to move, to read, to watch TV, to think. There was no part of me that was ready to die, but I understood why people gave up. I had felt how easy it would be just to slip away to the other side. Of course I wouldn't say that, or they would just add an antidepressant to the list of meds and call it a day. So I used concrete examples. I spent all day in bed. I could only go up the stairs once in a day, so I had to plan carefully. I was winded by the seventh step, and on and on. I described my fatigue by asking if they were familiar with Dementors from Harry Potter, the ghostly creatures that when creeping close enough to a person to steal their breath would then steal the very essence of their soul and leave their bodies behind as an empty shell.

The words "cumulative effects" had been mentioned by so many. Nurses even said it with a sympathetic smile. Those words terrified me. "Cumulative effects will kill me. My body can't handle more than this. I know it," I said adamantly. I was terrified mostly because I knew what was coming. I knew how bad it was, and the thought that it could and would get worse was impossible to fathom. The nurse listened, and she heard me. I know she did because I saw the tears pricking her eyes in understanding of my desperation.

Then Dr. S arrived and she agreed to dose down. She said she was already planning to do it based on my symptoms and our call the previous week. "The goal is to get you to the end, and if we have to adjust a few things here and there to do it, we can."

"So the reduction will keep it from getting worse?"

"It should. Most likely your experience for the next two rounds will be similar to this past one. You can use the tools that you have at your disposal. I can increase your prescription for Ativan, for example, as we have determined it helps with the heart palpitations, and most likely will help with other symptoms as well. That's what these drugs were made for. It's okay to use them in temporary circumstances like these. The most important thing is to keep going, to move forward."

I agreed, and the team all seemed relieved.

Chemotherapy is barbaric. There is no way around it. Even the surgeon admitted that we might look back at this treatment in the future and be appalled. Then he shrugged his shoulders and looked at me a bit sheepishly and said, "Right now this is the best we have." The oncologist, her RN, and everyone else I spoke to, continually referred to my particular treatment as "the gold standard" as if that special name made it something to aspire to instead of a horrible and potentially lethal cocktail of toxic pharmaceuticals. I was so sick of hearing the term. They might as well have said we're throwing everything and the kitchen sink at you because we have to cover all our bases. They all said, "You have to do this. You're too young not to." I had to accept it. I had to make peace, but it was by far the toughest choice I'd ever been faced with. Give up a year of my life or spend the rest of it in fear wishing I had. I chose to do what they told me, but I wasn't going to do it without giving all of them a hard time about it. Giving up a year of my life in exchange for a good chance at many more may seem worth it on paper, but living through the misery day by day changed the game.

It would have been easier to accept if it were a better-known issue. As far as breast cancer research had come, there were still so many un-resolved issues. Each treatment I would undertake—surgery, chemo-therapy, radiation, hormone blockers—would increase my survival and recurrence rate percentage, so I would do all of it, not knowing which therapy would help, which was unnecessary for me, and which could cripple me with side effects for the rest of my life. I would just do it because they thought/hoped/predicted that it would give me the best chance to live a long life. It was a head game as much as anything. It was like the feeling of vertigo I get when I lie on the grass staring into a deep blue sky...as if I could actually feel the gravity that holds me to the earth by a string.

Lea texted me.

"I think I'm going to out you on Facebook today. It seems like you could use the extra boost and know how much people love you. Everything will be fine. You can do this!"

A few minutes later I was notified that I was tagged in a post.

I clicked on the link and saw a photo that Lea had taken of us on the deck while she was here. Above it she had written, "Prayers, posi-tive thoughts, zen, whatever you've got. Aime my brave, tough sis is facing her third round of hard chemo today. It will be tough, but she can handle it. She is a bad ass ninja warrior in a fabulous wig."

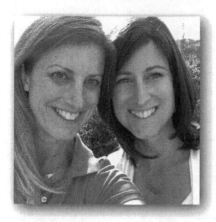

Say what you will about Facebook, but that post on that day might have saved my life. The love poured in from the friends that Lea and I have both collected throughout our lives, and the next few hours would have been a completely different experience without them. But if one more cheerful person told me that exercise cured fatigue, I was going to scratch their eyes out.

Week Six

Eventually I pulled through that round, which was much the same as round two—no better, but no worse—and the following week we were ready to move. Scott booked us into a hotel so the packers could get everything completely ready to go in one day, then we would move the next. We each packed a handful of things in our rollaway bags, which Scott loaded into the car, and then I dropped the kids off at school before the packers arrived. I camped out on the deck, soaking up the last few hours of the prized view of the canyon with the smell of eucalyptus wafting down over me while they went through the house like a hurricane wrapping and placing in crates everything that I hadn't given or thrown away. It's amazing how quickly a team of professionals can wrap up your life's possessions.

By lunchtime I knew the packers had it under control and drove to the cottage to check in with Shelley's contractors, who were helping put together the new loft beds for the kids and meet the utility crews. I pulled up to the cottage, and immediately a sense of calm washed over me. It was so green and quiet. The gardeners had just cut the wild spring grass around the house and blown the leaves away from the drive and walkway. I got out of my car and called hello to the contractors when I entered the house. Their voices echoed back from the kids' room, and I looked around. Everything was sparkling. The floors and windows had just been cleaned, the paint had been touched up, and light filtered through the glass doors that overlooked the patio and were framed by long, white, cotton panel drapes. Wandering into the kitchen, I saw a stash of goodies left by Shelley with a note.

"Just a few essentials from me and the girls to get you started. There are waters and beer for Scott in the fridge, and treats for Mav and…cat. Enjoy and welcome home! xoxo Shelley"

I checked in with the contractors, who had made great progress with the beds. The kids' room was shaping up to be adorable. Wesley's new bed was a half loft and was placed on top of his blue rug with boats around the edges. It had red and blue curtains that hung under the bed with windows and a little door, creating his own little play space where he planned to keep his Legos. Catherine's loft was much bigger, with a full bed and ladder over three sides of shelving and a desk. I could easily imagine her filling it with all her horse show ribbons, paintings, and favorite books, not to mention her own set of Legos that she still loved to play with.

For a split second I thought of our gracious old four-bedroom colonial currently occupied by tenants on the north shore of Boston but quickly put it out of my mind. We could do this. It helped to think about the fourteen hundred square feet being comparable to Manhattan with the added benefit of some outdoor space, and in this case it was quite a lot. Eight acres on Billionaire's Row in Woodside was the stuff of dreams for all but a very select few. And it was cute. It was a sweet little place, and we were lucky to be there. A number of things had had to line up to make it possible— Shelley being the broker, Scott closing his deal, and my being able to line up the help to make it happen. I knew we were there by the skin of our teeth, and I was grateful.

Scott took the afternoon shift to finish up with the packers while I got the kids from school and checked into the hotel. I promised them a swim in the pool if they finished their homework, so they got to work immediately, and I went into the bathroom to change my wig for a scarf before I could collapse on the freshly made bed beckoning me with its crisp white sheets and blanket.

Catherine followed me into the bathroom, and I warned her, "I'm going to take off my wig now, so you might want to give me some privacy for a minute." The wig was soft. Going for the real human hair had been a good call, but it felt like wearing a snug cap all the time. After wearing it all day, it felt a little hot and uncomfortable.

"No, I want to see." She smiled at me with mischief on her face.

"Are you sure? It's pretty weird." I asked her, not quite sure I was ready myself for anyone else to see.

"Yes, I really want to! It's not that big of a deal, Mama!"

Wesley, listening from the room like always, piped in, "It's okay, Mama, because I *don't* want to see!"

I relented and pulled off the hair, draping it over the angled mirror attached to the wall, and rubbed the little remaining bristles on my head while I crinkled up my nose. Catherine kept a good face, gave me a little smile, then left the room.

Wesley told me that she shuddered when she came out of the bathroom. She laughed and admitted it. "But it's okay, Mama. It's fine. I mean it."

With my soft silk scarf firmly in place, I collapsed onto the bed for an hour of oblivion. After the kids got their homework done, they pulled me down to the hotel pool. While watching them with one eye, I checked my phone and saw a text from Lauren.

"Hey! Would you be interested in grabbing pizza tonight with the kids at that good place by our house? And then possibly joining us to hang for the night?"

I was having trouble even lifting my hand to respond at that point so I just jotted out a quick few words. "Thanks so much for asking, but I'd better not. It's been a really long day and another tomorrow. Got to get through the move—it feels like a Herculean effort!"

"I'm sure! In the end it is all worth it ☺ xoxo"

I thought about it for a minute, that there was some alternate universe where a person might have the energy to meet friends for dinner in the middle of a move and chemo, and it sounded lovely. But I wasn't there. Not even close.

Moving day went off without a hitch, the beauty of hiring experts. Sometimes you can throw money at a problem, and as one of Scott's friends once said, "Movers are the most underpaid people in the world. I would pay them anything they asked to avoid doing the job myself."

I had mapped out where all the furniture would go with things that didn't fit being stored in the carport until we could find a place for them or put them in a storage pod. We had six movers and two trucks. As they stepped off the truck with each stack of crates or piece of furniture, I pointed them in various directions between the house, the shed, and the carport. Catherine watched my movements in fascination, "It's like you're a movie director!" she said, whizzing by on her newly unpacked scooter.

I laughed at her and said, "I've had a lot of practice!"

Scott spent the day alternating between running out for food and helping to shift the furniture around, and Wesley supervised the unpacking and careful placement of all of his Lego creations. Then at the end of the day we all collapsed on the couch together and ate a pizza dinner in our new home.

The next day while the kids were at school, I spent the time going back and forth between resting and unpacking, keeping up the sort of walk, run, walk pattern my Dad had taught us, saying, "You can go forever that way if you need to."

My deck chair had already found a new place under the shade of a graceful old water oak on the patio, and I would steal fifteen minutes of bliss at a time, staring up into the tree's heavy branches and listening to the sounds of the new space. There were so few houses within sight that the birds and animals that had taken up residence on the property dominated the soundscape. I noticed several woodpeckers flitting from tree to tree, and the occasional rustling from a squirrel. Fat little lizards squirmed their way around the hedges and paused, pumping up and down on their arms while they eyed me to determine how serious a threat I was.

I scooped up the kids after school, and the tires crushed the gravel as I swung the car into the driveway.

"Oh, look!" Catherine pointed out the deer curled up just a few feet away, his multi-horned rack up in watchful caution, but we didn't seem to bother him. The rest of the buck's family grazed peacefully on the dried grass on the other side of the drive, a couple of does and a baby young enough to still have spots on its back.

"Where is Maverick, sleeping on the job?" I pondered out loud, enjoying the deer but worrying that something might be wrong with him to let them come so close to the house. At that moment his great furry head burst up from the bushes under the great oak in front of the cottage. Blinking his eyes heavy from sleep, he shook his body in a quick quiver than ran down his back. He saw our car first and gave his tail a wag, then instantly tensed his body when he spotted the deer. He bounded over the bushes he had moments before been buried beneath and raced after the deer with an impressive speed that in contrast to his normal amble changed his look from polar bear to cheetah as he kicked dust up behind him. The kids whooped and cheered as we turned to watch a doe bound gracefully over the fence as Maverick chased the buck to the gate. Once the buck had passed through the gate, Maverick turned with record speed on a second doe pulling up the rear of the group and chased her until he was satisfied they were clearly off of our property. He slowly trotted back toward us, panting heavily but with a confident wag to his tail.

"Good boy, Maverick!" I rubbed his ears lightly. "You're doing such a good job protecting us from those scary deer." He grinned at me and plopped back down under the cover of the patio next to the front door with a loud grunt, huffing loudly in a self-righteous victory.

"Yeah, you got 'em, Mav. They'll definitely stay out of the yard until you go back to sleep," Wesley snickered.

The cottage was a slam dunk for Maverick at least, I thought, eyeing the stacks of crates that still needed to be unpacked. Actually we were all settling in well, and as much as I would have preferred not to move in the middle of chemo, it did seem to be a good fit. It was like a retreat, an extended vacation house where we got to live while we went on with our real lives.

I headed back to my bedroom, my shoulders letting go of some tension as I breathed a heavy sigh of relief and pulled my wig off.

Catherine had followed me and plopped down on my bed, watching me with a playful expression. "I wish I could take my hair off sometimes," she said with a giggle as I rubbed the stubble before I reached for my scarf. "I'll bet that feels pretty good."

"Actually, it does." I teased her back, flopping down beside her and pulling up my arms in a deep stretch. I looked up at the whitewashed wood-paneled ceiling with heavy crossbeams. The room was a tight squeeze for our king-sized bed, but it fit with a couple of feet to spare between the wall of built-ins that substituted for a closet and a decent-sized bathroom that I had been thrilled to see had a double sink and glass shower stall. Behind our bed was a wide window with a screen that we could open at night to listen to the frogs by the creek and let the fresh air blow through the room to the double doors three steps past the foot of the bed. There was also a fireplace squeezed into the corner of the room of which Scott had adopted the mantel to hold his baseball cap collection. It was a sweet place, and it was home, for now.

A couple of hours later I put Wesley to sleep in his new bed. We had devised a staggered bedtime routine so that he and Catherine wouldn't keep each other awake.

"So what do you think?" I asked, looking around while I leaned against the railing of his loft bed. "Is it okay sharing a room?" We had gotten most of the boxes unpacked and clearly defined a boy side and a girl side of the room.

He smiled his big gap-toothed grin and pulled the covers up around his chin, then stuck his thumbs up. "There are two reasons why I like it better." He put his thumbs down and held up two fingers. "First, my new bed is very cozy, and second, I am not alone."

"So you think it's better having Catherine in the room with you?" I asked, surprised to hear him admit it.

"Yes," he said. "I sleep better when there is someone else in the room, even if that person is Catherine."

I laughed and kissed his wet hair. "I get it."

I went to take my own shower, and the steam surrounded me as the water washed the day away. I lathered up my now shiny bald head with the new shampoo I had just gotten from Amazon after searching, "natural hair growth," for the promotion of healthy new hair growth. It said it right on the bottle. Watching the lather run down my belly and legs, I noticed the other hair that remained missing. Well, at least I don't have to shave, I thought, but I'd like to have a little back for some privacy.

I startled as I saw the door start to open through the glass shower walls.

"Stop!" I called, "I'm bald in here!"

"It's just me," Scott said as he pushed his way through the door. "I have to go to the bathroom."

"But I'm bald!" I cried.

"It's no big deal. I've seen it before."

I wanted to yell at him to get out, but he was right, it was no big deal. I hunched over anyway while my body shook, and I wept silently. I could see myself in the mirror through the steamed shower door, all yellow and pointy headed and scrawny huddled against the water stream. I looked like an alien. I didn't see anything of myself there, and I didn't want anyone else to see it either. It was the stuff of nightmares, and once I moved past this I didn't want any of us holding these images in our heads.

I was counting on the short term memory loss of Ativan and the chemo to help me forget, but I didn't know how long these images would be burned into Scott's brain. How could he ever find me attractive or God forbid sexy after seeing this thing that lived underneath?

That night he came in the room after I was already in bed with my sleeping cap on. He snuggled up to me and took it off, rubbing my head. "It's okay," he whispered. "I still think you're beautiful. It's going to grow back. It will all be okay." He ran his hands down my sides and gave my butt a pat the way I always loved. I cried again and melted into him as we fell asleep with his big protective arms wrapped around me.

CHAPTER 18

❧

I Can Be Your Uber
May—Week Seven

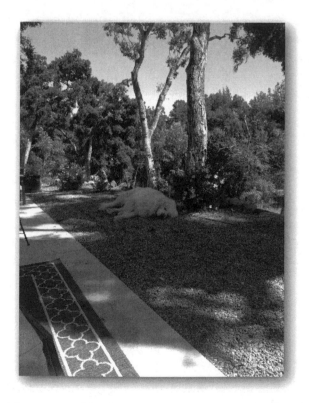

Aime: Would you mind picking me up tomorrow before lunch?
I am going to uber it to Stanford right after ☺

Shelley: I can do that! I can also be your uber if you like. Just don't write any bad reviews of me… I have an apt in Los Altos Hills at 8:45 and then have great flexibility until 4.
Aime: That would be wonderful! I'm nervous about tomorrow so looking forward to hanging with you in the am!!
Shelley: Let's do it! I will calm your nerves. Can I ply you with alcohol?
Aime: I wish! No alcohol until after chemo ☹
Shelley: I will bore you with real estate stories.
Shelley: Oh wait, I will tell you about the time Jim chased a raccoon out of the house when he was naked.
Aime: That would not be boring! Chased a raccoon? That's quite a visual!
Shelley: Yes! Tell me about it…the neighbors moved a few months after
Aime: I would love to hear no-names-attached Silicon Valley real estate stories!! Haha!
Shelley: I got the stories! Look forward to seeing you.
Aime: Me too!!

I HAD BEEN unpacking and settling into the new cottage at a fever pitch the past few days so that by the fourth round I would have things generally in place. It was exhausting, but the move was giving me busy work and keeping my mind off my own physical issues in a way that seemed to be serving me well, and I was so happy to be back in the country again.

We had set up the outdoor furniture in the back of the house on a concrete patio that connected our bedroom and the living room to the kitchen with a series of double doors. It overlooked the back slope of the yard that stretched down toward a creek that ran along the side of the property and under a wooden bridge to the street. Catherine had been the first to notice that the bridge had been made for the horse trail that connected many of the barns in Woodside, so every day we heard the clomp clomping of their heavy hooves as they made their way over the bridge and through the end of the yard.

My life had been drastically simplified by the shorter commutes to school and Stanford, and our downsizing of furniture and assorted things made the revolving tasks of the household much easier to tackle. A bonus had been Maverick no longer requiring twice-a-day walks because he had so much space to roam, and chasing deer and barking at passing horses kept him gleefully occupied.

The previous months had seen a steady spiral out of control, but I finally felt as if things were settling down. We had responded to the chaos, we had made some changes, and they were working. The simplicity of it all was astonishing.

Shelley picked me up the next day and we drove the minute and a half to the Woodside Bakery in the Woodside town center. Shelley would call it quintessential Woodside, a sweet little neighborhood place, but it was definitely the realm of the local "ladies who lunch."

We were shown to a booth inside and settled in. Shelley always took a few minutes to warm up. Her natural state was highly professional and polished, and I made it my mission to wear her down until she relaxed with me.

"My mother enjoyed meeting you at Easter," Shelley said as she pulled the crisp white napkin onto her lap. "She said she liked your East Coast preppie look. She approves."

I felt a wistful pang when she mentioned her mother, as always, thinking of my own and what she might have said about the weekend, or my dress, or my wig. I always thought of her in Carmel because she and Dad had come out for our first Thanksgiving in California, and we had spent it there.

We had met up with Jackie's family, and the kids were restless to get down to the beach. We all rolled our eyes at Mom as she stopped in probably fifteen stores looking for a scarf until she found just the perfect one—a cranberry red finely woven linen cotton blend that she wrapped loosely around her neck, letting the ends float free in the ocean breeze. It complemented her dark hair sprinkled with silver strands perfectly and brought out a little color in her cheeks. She wore it proudly for the rest of the weekend. I never thought that those would be some of our last moments together. I would have stayed with her, shopped with her, talked to her about nonsense all day, all week, for as long as I could if I'd known.

I smiled at Shelley and replied, "That's so sweet. It's wonderful you have her so close."

"It's a mixed blessing," she said as she tilted her head to the right.

"Family," I said. "But really. I'm so glad we could do this. I'm a little nervous about going in today. It's my last heavy chemo, and it's nice to have the distraction beforehand. Lovely company and a good meal before I'm nauseated for another week."

"I'm happy to be here. Anything you need," Shelley replied.

We chatted through lunch about summer plans and other things before the conversation moved back to the event of the day.

"So is Scott going with you to the doctor?"

I was slightly puzzled by the question. "No, should he? I'd rather him spend the energy taking care of us on my down days when I really need him. Because then I really need him. Today is just a mental issue." I smiled, trying to shrug it off. I did see other couples together and sometimes family members accompanying patients into the offices, but they were always so much older. They looked so much more helpless than I was, like they needed someone to take care of them. On most days I took great pride in the fact that I did not. I relished in the somewhat normal energy level that I had finally bounced back to. That day I could walk, drive, brush my teeth and get dressed all by myself, and damn it, I would. Because I knew by the next day the energy I enjoyed would be gone again.

The last thing I wanted was for Scott to leave work again just to sit with me in one of countless waiting rooms to hear a fifteen-minute conversation, which I could easily relay to him that night when he came home with dinner. I had to be unproductive for the time being, but I needed him to get his shit done, and a lot of mine too.

I checked the time on my phone. "Oh shoot."

Shelley asked, "Time to go?" and waved for our check.

I nodded. "Are you sure you don't mind taking me in?"

"Aime, it's what I do. Drive around all day. It's in my triangle, anyway. Don't give it a second thought. I'm your new Uber."

I laughed. "Thanks."

Uber had been a useful tool these past few weeks, but it had inevitably produced awkward moments. The drivers never failed to comment on the neighborhood, how they rarely got to drive on the country roads and were often surprised at how close they were to the hustle and bustle across the interstate even though they felt miles away. They often asked me what I was doing, expecting me to talk about lunch with friends or some other kind of pleasant outing, and I would vaguely reply that I had a doctor's appointment. And always, as I directed them to the building clearly marked Women's Cancer Center, they quit talking.

Shelley pulled into the circular drive of the cancer center, and suddenly I remembered to take my Ativan. The nurses had said I should start taking it before these heavy chemo sessions to make them easier to manage. I searched through my purse, hoping I had remembered the bottle.

"What are you looking for?" Shelley asked.

"Um. I think I forgot my Ativan." I looked up and from her shift in expression I knew she must have seen the worry on my face. "I take it for anxiety on chemo days." I kept digging through my purse, hoping it would miraculously appear. "Maybe Scott could go home and get it," I said, my voice trailing off.

"Aime, let me get it for you," she said.

"Oh, that's so sweet. No, really. I'll call Scott." I admonished myself for forgetting, cringing at the thought of sending Shelley back to my house and having to rummage through my bathroom searching for the bottle I had carelessly left behind.

"Aime, let me do it. Now that you're back in Woodside I just have to run up the hill and back. Scott doesn't have to leave work. I could be back in twenty minutes."

"Oh, no, it's too much." I said, reluctant to take up any more of her time when she'd already spent the past two hours with me.

"Aime," Shelley touched my arm and held my gaze. "It's no bother at all. It's just a few minutes to and from your house. Let me take care of it."

Finally I conceded and was overcome with relief. She was right. She had the time, and I needed the help. "Okay," I said and handed her my house key.

"Okay." She smiled, gave me a quick hug, and said, "I'll be right back."

I checked in and was brought back to the exam room early, then Shelley texted:

Shelley: turning on Pasteur
Aime: oh shoot—I'm in the drs office. Maybe I need you to come in and keep me company for a while? Do you mind park-ing for a bit?
Shelley: at red light. Omg. Leaving your place I saw 6 blue birds! Yes will park
Aime: Really? Good signs, right?
Shelley: Yes! And you brought me amazing luck. Got a call from agent who saw my car in the Woodside parking lot. Has new listing perfect for my client!
Shelley: Where do I go?

At that point a nurse had come in and I reluctantly put away my phone, hoping Shelley would be able to find me. This was a big ask. I was sure when she offered to give me a ride to Stanford, she hadn't committed to staying for hours.

After a few minutes there was a knock on the exam room door. I heard a quick conversation with the nurse and she asked, "Is it okay for your friend to come in? She wanted me to ask."

"Of course. Hi!" I smiled as Shelley floated in like an exotic butterfly, brightly lighting up the otherwise bland room.

"Oh, sorry," she said as she breezed in holding out two medicine bottles. "Is it okay for me to come in? I have your medicine. I brought everything I could find, just in case you need anything else today." She rattled the bottles and handed them to me.

"Thank you so much. That was so sweet of you!"

The nurse looked at Shelley curiously, and I introduced them.

"So do you want me to stay? I left my car with the valet and have an open afternoon, so I can stay and keep you company if you want."

"Well, since you're here, sure!"

Shelley settled herself down in one of the chairs next to the exam table while the nurse excused herself and told us Dr. S would be in shortly. The solitary waiting time that I normally had in the office turned into an extension of our lunch conversation and seemed just as light.

When Dr. S came in, I introduced them, saying, "I brought along a friend today. We're having an extended lunch date."

Dr. S laughed, and they exchanged a few pleasantries before we got down to business. Shelley stared intently at her phone, giving me a version of privacy while I ran down the list of symptoms I continued to have. My main problems continued to be fatigue, but I was starting to lose some real weight by then, and I tried to explain the difference I could see in my skin and my overall appearance.

"My eyes look so tired, and my skin is yellow and seems so thin and almost wrinkly," I said.

Dr. S looked me over. "You seem okay to me. All of this is to be expected. If you looked totally normal I would suspect that you weren't actually being given the right medicines."

I gave her a courtesy smile for the little joke, but continued, feeling that she needed to have a more accurate reference. "I just don't even look like myself anymore. I can try to dress myself up with makeup, but I can really tell the difference." I looked at Shelley and wondered if she could be the outside voice that would be able to verify the change in my appearance. "Shelley, don't I look totally different?"

Shelley looked up from her phone with a startled look, then shook her head and said, "I think you look beautiful."

It was so sweet and unexpected that it caught me by surprise. "I pay her to say that," I said. "I pay her with lunch and green tea lemonades." I let out a peel of laughter while Shelley and Dr. S joined me in relief. We wrapped up and walked over to the infusion center together.

Not just anyone can drop into a chemo treatment—most people, even cheerful Laura, preferred to do the day alone. I never really thought about wanting or needing company until the nurse had said, "All by yourself today?" as in "Table for one?" the previous round. The nurses provide good comfort and company, so I would never want anyone just sitting in with me because they didn't want me to be alone or because they felt obligated to be there. It's not the place for a casual friend or acquaintance. But somehow Shelley fit in beautifully.

CHAPTER 19

❧

What I Missed Week Eight

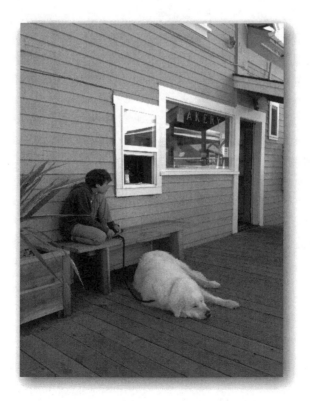

AFTER MY FOURTH and final round of the AC chemo, I was left battered and beaten but looking ahead toward the next phase, twelve weeks of Taxol chemotherapy, which I had been told and sold would be easier.

I was counting on it. I needed it to be that way so badly. I was physically and emotionally worn out from the chemo, our move, and my mounting task list, but finally a reprieve seemed to be in sight. It was the end of the school year, and Catherine was nearing her graduation from Episcopal School. The school had a tradition of showcasing all of the special projects that the students had completed throughout the year in one big night called SMARTS night, standing for Science, Music and ART. In previous years I had looked forward to that night, to finally see what they had been working so hard on, and they were always so proud to show off their accomplishments. But that year it fell too close to the last AC round, and I didn't bounce back quickly enough. Scott took the kids alone, and I was devastated to have to miss it. Just one more thing, one more moment, one more night ripped away from me. Scott texted me photos of the kids smiling proudly by their favorite displays.

When they got home, the kids ran in to tell me about their night while Scott rustled around in the new kitchen. Once he had gotten the kids going on their bedtime routine, he checked in on me. "Shelley gave us some pizza if you can eat anything," he said. "It's warming up now."

I thought for a moment and was relieved when my stomach didn't turn. "I'll try a slice. How did it go tonight?" I got up and followed him into the kitchen.

He filled me in on the projects the kids had each presented, pausing while he pulled the pizza out of the oven. "Let's eat outside," he said. "It's nice out."

I grabbed a throw blanket from the couch and wrapped it around me to create a cocoon against the cool night air. Scott put the pizza on the side table between our two chairs and moved his speakers outside, turning on a mellow live My Morning Jacket recording.

The music soothed me, as he knew it would. It spoke of our shared history, the shows we had seen together, the points where our tastes matched, and the many hours we had spent like this. I sank into the chair, pulling the thick fuzzy fleece around my chin, and gazed up at the night sky, dizzy with stars, framed by the branches of the oak.

We had been through rough patches before, and he always tended to handle them the same way. To work harder. He saw that as his contribution, the best way he could help, but I hoped that he would realize that what we all really wanted from him was to be with us. I knew it went against all of his instincts, but those previous couple of months he hadn't had a choice, and I think in ways it was good for us.

A couple of days later, Catherine's entire class presented movies they had each made individually to illustrate a historical event or person they had learned about. I came in late and sat in one of the back rows of chairs set up in the darkened library and watched seventeen movies before Catherine's came on. She had chosen a female doctor from the 1800s named Elizabeth Blackwell. I felt a shiver of nerves as she walked up to the front of the room. I had no idea what she would present. I hadn't seen her work on any of it. She took the microphone from a classmate and stood poised in front of all the parents and her peers and talked about the impact of this woman's life in a clear and meaningful way. She was growing before my eyes, and I was missing it.

There were a few more presentations after hers and then the group moved to the classroom to admire the children's presentation boards and to learn more about their work. We were asked to walk through all of them, but I knew I couldn't do it. I was so weak by then that taking more than a few steps left me winded. The classroom was hot and stuffy, and I felt my chest constricting in gasps for air.

One of Catherine's friend's mothers stood next to us and reached out to touch my shoulder with a careful pat. She and her husband peered anxiously at me then she said, "That's a pretty dress you have on."

I smiled weakly in response and looked down at what had been one of my favorite summer dresses swimming around my emaciated body. I could see the concern in their eyes. They tried graciously to hide it, but what I saw reflected to me was shock and pity.

Catherine's teacher checked in with me and offered me a seat in the other room, but the heat and the crowd were stifling. I hugged Catherine and told her how proud I was of her and asked her if she was okay with my leaving. She said she was fine and I scampered out, escaping to my car for a few minutes of rest.

An hour later, I was back at school waiting in the carpool line with the air conditioner and engine running. I knew I was wasting gas and contributing to global warming by idling my car, but it was over ninety degrees in the sun, and I needed to breathe.

Lauren parked her car nearby and bounced over toward me, her long red ponytail swinging behind her while she tugged her T-shirt down over her yoga pants. I rolled down the window as she waved at me, a rush of hot air flooding the car.

"Hi!" she said. "How's it going? It's so hot out, right?"

"Oh, I know. I just couldn't walk in today."

"So how's it going? You're done with the heavy chemo, right?"

"I am. Just recovering before I start Taxol next week. Twelve more weeks of something new, but they say it should be easier."

"Well, let me know if you're up for a walk or something."

"Oh, thanks, but I don't think I'm quite ready for that yet. It's taking all of my energy to get the new house settled and keep up with the things I have to do for the kids." The thought of having to exercise in this heat with my wig on distracted me for a minute, and I had to refocus to keep my smile plastered. "So how are things with you?"

"Oh, they're good. I'm just so busy..." she then went through a barrage of endless activities that she had become involved with, all of which were having their big end-of-the-year celebrations/presentations/performances and what have you. My eyes glazed over while I tried to keep the smile on my face. She finally finished with a loud exaggerated exhale and a wipe of her brow, "Just the typical end-of-the-year craziness, you know?"

"Yeah."

"Well, I'd better run and get Elizabeth. Take care, okay?"

"Okay, you too." I rolled up the window and adjusted the air vents toward my face. It struck me that everything she was complaining about was a choice she had made, and most of it was optional. Girl Scouts, ballet, choir, the litany of extracurriculars. The merry-go-round of the overachieving mom that I was happy I had stepped off of if only to give me a moment to step back and see what it really looked like. We wanted to do all of this to benefit our children, but was it really helping them? Was keeping them over-scheduled and loaded up with structured activities good for them or for us? I was beginning to think it was good for nobody.

Weeks Nine and Ten

I had been advised that the issues that might come up with Taxol were allergic reaction, which would present within the first thirty minutes of infusion if it were a problem, and then an adjustment week while my body was still processing the Adriamycin and Cytoxan and adjusting to the influx of Taxol. Then I was supposed to feel some relief for the first several weeks of Taxol until eventually I felt the cumulative effects toward the end. Those fucking cumulative effects. But I focused on the task at hand, and that was starting and adjusting to Taxol. My new chemotherapy. My new companion drug for the next twelve weeks.

I had round one of Taxol the Thursday before Memorial Day. I was pumped with steroids and Benadryl to avoid allergic reactions and made it through the infusion smoothly. The following few days passed in a flu-like haze of fatigue and achy bones. My main complaints were neuropathy in my hands, which left them itchy, red, and swollen with numb fingertips; intense flashes of bone pain, which invariably started up in the afternoons as soon as my body needed a rest; and on-and-off head rushes, like those I had felt on my heavy chemo days. My cognitive function had improved, though, and while the noise of the television was grating to me, I plowed through hours of historical romance novels while my body rested. It was the literary version of candy for my brain.

Then just one week later, I went in for Taxol Two. It was hard to get my head around going back after just a week, but I knew that things were feeling different, a little better, and I was ready to move on through the motions.

I went through the blood test, the waiting, and the exam routine, and then Dr. S came in to ask how I was.

"I think this is a lot better so far," I said, carefully upbeat. "I was tired and achy, but I'm starting to feel better, I think." I looked down at my notes and rattled off the rundown. She laughed as I ended with my ability to binge read light novels. "Hey, it's all informative, right? I'm sure most people don't have you judge their cognitive abilities based on their evening reading, do they?"

"No, they don't. You're enlightening me in all kinds of ways, Aime. All right, let me see your hands." She reached out to me with both hands and took mine in hers, looking at my fingernails and the tips of my fingers to judge the neuropathy, a condition that causes the fingertips and toes to develop a numb, tingling sensation that could become permanent.

"I'm going to take you down a little bit. I think we've established that works best for you and should help with the numbness."

"Okay, let's do it then," I agreed, happy with news of an approved dose-down. I went over to the infusion center with a lighter step. Just two more rounds, then we would take extra days in between rounds to switch the schedule from Thursdays to Tuesdays for the rest of the summer. Switching in June also gave me the benefit of having five extra days to rest around Catherine's graduation, and I looked forward to it like an oasis in the desert. Scott's parents were coming to town and had offered to treat us to a weekend in Carmel Valley. Just holding onto the thought of a long weekend away got me through a lot of bad moments.

Week Eleven

Shelley cruised into the infusion center holding two venti green tea lemonades.

"You've got me hooked on these things," she grinned and handed one to me. I was already attached to the IV and settled into the reclining chair, having scoped out a prime seat by the window.

Shelley flipped her sunglasses up on her head and pulled over a chair. She pulled out a magazine to look at and thumbed through it for a minute.

"So, have you spent any time considering your fall look?"

I laughed in response, and she said, "No, seriously! You might have a cropped new cut by then, and I'm seeing you dressing it up with a leather moto jacket or something. Because you'll be showing everyone what a *bad ass* you are." She whispered the "bad ass," giving a quick glance to either side as if to check for children.

"Now that you mention it, I have thought about sporting a new pixie and how on earth I'll make that work." I shook my head because it wasn't a habit of mine to create a look for the season, but in actuality, I probably would this year to overcompensate for a seriously drastic hair style. "But I was thinking more Audrey Hepburn or Julie Andrews than Grace Jones. You know, cuffed skinny jeans, little flats and a boat neck sweater with wayfarer sunglasses."

"Hmmm." She nodded. "That's one way to go. But I think you should put some more thought into a moto jacket."

I snickered at her and leaned back in the seat. From anyone else the conversation might have irritated me, but somehow Shelley pulled off the most outrageous statements with humor. She would say something ridiculous and then just before my eyebrows went up in question, she would laugh about it, knowing how it sounded but not really caring that much.

Gradually we moved off fall fashion and on to catching up about the other girls.

"Have you heard from Lauren?" Shelley asked.

"Just a few text exchanges. She asked me to meet her to walk a couple of times, but it's always on the worst day and I haven't been able to go."

"Yes, she seemed pretty concerned about you the other day, but I told her I've been seeing you pretty often and you seemed fine."

"That's strange." I puzzled on that for a minute. "She hasn't even really talked to me lately other than a couple of texts that I answered.

"I don't know." Shelley waved her hand as if to shoo the disruption away. "I think it was something about wanting to add more dates to the Meal Train thing."

I sighed. "I know. The Meal Train was so nice, and it was so sweet of everyone to pitch in like that. But by now I've got things figured out better. Everyone took a turn and brought a meal, and I don't think they need to do it anymore."

"I was wondering about that," she said. "I wasn't sure if I would like that or not, either."

"It's really very nice of everyone, so I hate to even criticize it at all." I paused and tried to think of how to frame the issue. "It's just that sometimes it's better to organize our own meals. That way we know when it will be there, what it will be, and it's not lasagna."

Shelley laughed, "That's right. I guess everyone wants to make a big lasagna for you, but how many times can you eat that?"

"Once a month or once every six months." I laughed. "The kids don't even really like it. But then I feel so bad. I know how much it took for someone to go to the trouble to make something for us and drive it over in the busiest part of the day when the kids need to get home to do their homework and be fed themselves. And some people did just the perfect thing at the perfect time. So I really did love it. It was so sweet of everyone, but I think they've done enough. I'm sorry if it hurts Lauren's feelings, but if I don't need it..." I let the sentence trail off and looked away.

When people dropped by loads of food in containers that needed to be promptly cleaned and returned, they had no idea that some days just getting to the sink took an enormous amount of effort. And so following complicated instructions or having too many pieces to a meal or having way too much food that needed to be transferred to containers and stuffed into my overflowing freezer was overwhelming me. I wanted to cry and kiss the person who gave me simple serving size portions in disposable containers. It seemed so easy, but it wasn't and I was too tired to communicate my needs and too reluctant to give instructions to someone who was giving me a gift of their time and energy.

"I get it." Shelley nodded enthusiastically. "That's why I bring you green tea lemonades. I know exactly what you want and how to get it!"

I picked up the clear plastic cup from the table beside me. It was wet with condensation and filled with the sweet gold elixir I had come to love. "You are so right," I said and took a long sip. I was still puzzling over Lauren being so concerned about me. It seemed like she would have said something to me if she really was.

"So here's some news," I said. "Dr. S gave me the all clear to book our Alaska trip today."

"That's wonderful!" Shelley said, her eyes widening while her head bobbed up and down. "Alaska?"

"Yes, originally we wanted to go up to Victoria Island in British Columbia, but that was sort of a high energy trip, so Scott found an Alaskan cruise that does a lot of the same stuff."

"What sort of stuff do you do in Alaska?"

"There's a ton to do, but I don't know how much energy I'll have at that point, so being on a cruise I can just hang out on the deck and take in the beautiful mountains and glaciers over the water while Scott and the kids hike and kayak."

Shelley had started wrinkling her nose at the idea, and I laughed. "What, you don't like an outdoorsy vacation?"

"If by outdoorsy you mean walking on the beach barefoot, then yes. But I'm not sure I would go quite so far as Alaska."

I laughed. "Suit yourself. I'll say hi to the whales for you." I couldn't imagine anything better. The cool fresh air would be a welcome relief from the summer heat I was not able to tolerate anymore, and with just an hour flight to Seattle, we could hop on the boat and then spend a week having all of our needs taken care of. We could sleep in every day, play as much or as little as we wanted, and most heavenly, not have to cook or organize a single meal.

I shifted, relaxing back in my chair. "So back to appearances for a minute. Tell me the truth. What do you think of the lashes?" My eyelashes had recently started falling out, so I had been playing with false ones.

"Let me see." She leaned in closer to me and studied my eyes as I opened and closed them to give her a better look.

"They look great," she replied, still closely observing me. "Very natural."

"Thanks," I said, choosing to believe her. "I've been working on them I tried a bunch of different kinds and settled on the individual lashes. I think I'm getting the hang of it. I'm sort of liking the heavy lash look. Maybe I'll keep it, even when my lashes grow back, now that I know how."

"And why shouldn't you?"

Scott rushed in toward the end of the infusion, sweating from the walk from the garage he must have taken at a run.

"Sorry, I'm late," he said. "I got hung up."

"No worries," I said. "Shelley was able to keep me company again."

He kissed Shelley hello, and then looked around frazzled and confused for a place to sit down. Shelley got up and found him a chair and table for his laptop, then settled herself back down next to me to continue our girl talk. Scott tried politely to listen in, eventually giving way to the pull of work emails until my infusion was done and we were released to go home.

CHAPTER 20

❦

Graduation
June—Week Twelve

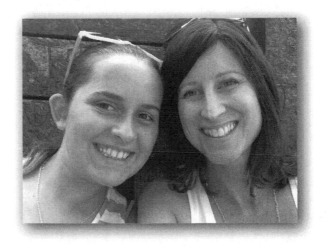

CATHERINE'S FIFTH GRADE graduation came and Scott's parents arrived from Boston. I used some precious energy to shop with Catherine for a new dress and got her first pair of low heels, which had to be purchased in the adult section of Nordstrom when we discovered that her feet had grown to the same size seven as my own. She looked beautiful in a gauzy mint green chevron print dress tied with a ribbon around the high part of her waist. Her normally free-flowing blond beach waves were blown out straight with a few soft curls around the ends, and she proudly wore the new silver Tiffany bracelet we had given her the night before.

I had been nervous for Scott's parents to see me. I knew that I looked drastically different at that point; I had seen it on the faces of people around me. I had caught my reflection in store windows and found myself unrecognizable, so skinny with yellow skin and a wig and fake eyelashes. But when everyone met at our house for dinner, it was all as it should be. They both hugged me and said I looked well. Their presence seemed to make Catherine's day into a much more important event, and we were all so glad to be able to mark the milestone together.

They graciously offered to stay in a nearby hotel, so we all met up the next morning for the graduation day. The ceremony was at eleven in the morning and I met Scott and his parents outside of the chapel, where the families gathered to wait for the children to go in. We all beamed with pride as the graduating fifth graders marched past us with dignity and serious faces, each preparing for the speech that they would give. The program was brief, allowing most of the time for the children to speak. It was a time-honored tradition of the school that each child had a moment to reflect on their elementary school years before they moved on.

Catherine had not shared her speech with us beforehand, and as she walked to the podium and adjusted the microphone, my heart was in my chest and I held my breath. Her calm, clear voice filled the chapel with a purity that only a child's voice can.

"Episcopal School has taught me and prepared me for the future. From social studies to PE, I have learned, grown and I have become a butterfly. When I came to Episcopal School in the beginning of third grade, I was only an egg waiting to go to my next stage in life. Soon I met my class and they welcomed me in with open arms. In fourth grade, I was more used to my class, and I was a caterpillar, learning and growing quickly. Then finally the fifth grade, which was my pupa stage and holds most of my favorite memories from Episcopal. My teachers and my class helped me to be who I am.

As I say goodbye to Episcopal School, I feel I have grown into a beautiful butterfly ready to take flight because of all the support I received from my teachers, my parents and my friends. Thank you."

My eyes welled up and I leaned my head against Scott's shoulder. Jackie and Shelley sat within sight to my right, and as everyone clapped politely, Jackie gave me a wink and a grin, tears welling in her own eyes, while Shelley beamed at me.

At the close of the ceremony all of the children in the school sang "Until we meet again." There is a special magic that comes from children's voices blending together in their high pitch the old and often-sung words from the hymnal. As we walked out to the courtyard, many people were wiping their eyes.

We were guided to create two lines of people, leaving an open pathway for the graduates to walk through, ending with a large arc of balloons that swung gently with the breeze. Containers of soap bubbles were passed out and adults were turned into children, blowing a steady stream of iridescent spheres down onto the heads of the proud fifth graders. Catherine spotted me in the crowd, then looked away quickly, her eyes straight ahead. She put her best Mona Lisa smile on as she saw me lift my phone for a photo. Another milestone. Another passage.

Weeks passed and I fell into a routine between weekly chemo treatments. I gradually started to feel a little better, reading a lot and sleeping in, spending a lot of time on my outdoor lounge chair under my favorite tree, the ancient water oak that graced me with its shade for the better part of the day. I started journaling and writing to keep track of what I was going through. Somehow I knew that if I didn't write it down I would forget it. I had three journals, one I used to rant and rave, feeling free to express my fears and details of my physical condition, and the other two for Catherine and Wesley. Those journals read like a series of love letters in which I shared my favorite memories with each of them and little traits I appreciated in them. Those pages I could only write a few of at a time before I would dissolve into tears.

I thought wistfully that something like yoga would feel soothing. The cancer center offered free classes in Palo Alto, but it always felt like it used too many of my fleeting and very valuable resources to get there, and I couldn't imagine doing the poses and keeping my head covered with my wig. So I let it pass, along with so many other things I had gotten used to giving up.

Scott was spending a lot of time planning our Alaska trip, which was a sign to me that the pressure was getting to him. I had always been able to tell when he was stressed at work because he would email me during the day asking what I thought about this or that hotel or activity for an upcoming trip. He once told me that one of the things that made his work bearable was that it allowed him to be able to travel when he needed to. It was always with careful planning, and on a budget, but I got it. It was something he really loved to do, and I couldn't deny that I enjoyed the benefits too. I was always just along for the ride on whatever the latest adventure he cooked up was. Since we had been in California we had been exploring the West Coast bit by bit. And now looking forward to Alaska was like a beacon in the storm. We planned it for the week after my last chemo treatment. It was our saying that if we could get to there, it would all be okay. So Scott planned it, and I eagerly read all the excursion descriptions and trip highlights he showed me. And together we counted down the days. To the end of chemo, and to Alaska.

Week Thirteen

Shelley: Hi There. How are you feeling today? What time to meet tomorrow and where for lunch? I can pick you up.

Aime: Do you want to just go somewhere here to make it easier? Or I can uber it to Palo Alto and do calafia, but I'll bet you're done with that!!! And thank you for the pick up offer!!

Shelley: What time is your first appointment? I am so excited to jet up from downtown Menlo to pick you up! Calafia does open at 11 which may be helpful. Bucks and Bakery always good. Any interesting restaurants at Stanford?

Aime: First apt is 1, there is that place in the Stanford barn cant remember the name, but it's really good

Shelley: Is it tootsie's?

Aime: That's it!

Shelley: Those are Lauren's friends and they donated to the benefit. I have been meaning to try it.

Aime: Sounds like a plan then! Should we ask Lauren to join us?

Shelley: That's a great idea. Do you want to reach out to her?

Aime: I will ☺

Then I texted Lauren:

Aime: Hi there! How's your summer? Any chance you can join me and Shelley for lunch on Thursday at Tootsies? Would love to see you and catch up!

Lauren: What time?

Aime: 11:30

After waiting for a while with no response from Lauren, I checked back in with Shelley.

Aime: I asked Lauren. She seems to be evaluating (tongue out)

Shelley: Checking her schedule I guess

A couple of hours later the response from Lauren finally came.

Lauren: I'm sorry, I can't. Have fun!

Later Shelley and I caught back up about it.

Shelley: Did Lauren get back to you re lunch?

Aime: She said she's busy?

Shelley: More food for us

Aime: Yes ☺ I think something scandalous is going on ;) or maybe it's all these romance novels I've been reading!

I was thrown off by Lauren's blunt refusal of our lunch invitation and started worrying, as I was apt to do. Was there something wrong? Had I said something? I asked Shelley about it, because I knew she and Lauren had remained close, and she agreed that it did seem odd but was reluctant to offer any excuses. So I talked to Jackie about it when we met up at the pool the next afternoon. By then my confusion was turning into an annoyance.

We were having a heat wave and we had escaped the un-air-conditioned cottage to our athletic club pool. I hid under an umbrella and wanted to dive into the pool to cool down, but with my wig I couldn't, so instead I watched longingly as the kids splashed and played and I sipped ice water, still thanking my lucky stars that at least we had a place to go.

"I'm not really sure what happened," I went on, after I had explained the whole situation to Jackie. We watched from the chairs under the shade of a huge blue umbrella as the kids chased each other with water guns. "I mean, I haven't reached out in a while, but I think I have a pretty good excuse. Surely she hasn't been offended in some way, do you think?"

Jackie smoothed her hair back and adjusted her sunglasses, "Yeah, I'm not really sure, either. First of all, I don't think it's your responsibility to be keeping up with people right now. That's our job as your friends and the people who love you. I do seem to remember her putting a lot of effort into the Meal Train thing and being a little hurt when you wanted to give it up."

"Oh, the Meal Train." I shook my head, remembering Shelley's earlier mention of it. "Yes, it was really nice when it happened, after the surgery and during the heavy chemo, but I remember it sort of playing out once everyone in the class had brought a meal, and by then I started not to need it as much." I tried to remember what I might have said to Lauren about it, and why she might be taking it so personally.

"I don't know." Jackie shook her head. Her light brown hair brushed her jawline while the corners of her mouth turned down. "My only guess is that she really wanted a role, and when you took it away from her, it hurt her feelings. I'm not saying it makes any sense. I'm just saying that's what she might be thinking." She laughed a little. "But seriously, none of this should worry you for a minute. The only thing you need to be thinking of is getting yourself better, and it's our job to listen to what you need and help you where we can."

"Oh my gosh, it sounds like I've been so ungrateful! I never meant to be that way about it. It was so nice for people to want to reach out and help. After a while it was just enough."

"Aime, noooooo." She drew out the word in her signature two syllables. "Everyone knows how appreciative you have been! You have told us all! We all just wanted to do something for you, and we did, and now it's done and that's that!" She punctuated her last sentence, punching a polished fingernail onto my lounge chair beside my stretched out leg.

We fell into silence for a moment, keeping one eye on the battle between the kids that had moved on to include kickboards. Then Jackie spoke out again. "I have this bifurcation theory of friends, and it's really helped me out in situations like this."

"Yeah," I nodded. "Wait, did you just say bifurcation? Bifurcation of friends?"

"Hah!" She laughed loudly and I joined her.

I had only heard the term in what I considered "corporate speak" by Scott and others in networking situations.

"Please explain the theory!" I said.

"So bifurcation means that you are putting things into separate categories, or pods, right? So there are different categories of friends, and it's helpful to know which category each friend belongs in. One is for people you barely know, one is for work friends or school friends, another one for closer acquaintances, and then at the core you have your very close friends. Sometimes you have to move people from one to another once you get to know them better, but it's okay because they still have a place in your life. Not everyone can be the same kind of friend. Not like you, my dear."

We smiled at each other, mutually grateful for the level we each maintained in the other's life. I had known Jackie for three years at that point, but it felt like I had known her all my life. Lauren and even Shelley had always struck me as these bright, shiny things, impossibly tall, thin, and always so current- wearing the latest styles and always knowing the trending topic of the day. Somehow they felt more like a challenge to me. I adored them both, but it was different than the way Jackie seemed like the combination of a comrade at arms and a sister.

"That makes a lot of sense. I like the bifurcation theory. It's not personal, and I can't expect people to fit into categories that they shouldn't. In the center of things I guess there is one main category. That's what my mom used to call ya-yas. From that book she loved." I said.

"Exactly! In your whole life you might have only five or ten ya-yas, and that's if you're lucky." Jackie sat back and adjusted her dark framed sunglasses against the glare. "Now how about an Arnold Palmer?"

A few minutes later she came back with two clear plastic cups, an Arnold Palmer for me and a generous pour of white wine for herself.

"Cheers," she clinked cup against mine.

"Cheers," I said. "I'm jealous of your wine, but not jealous enough to try some yet. Oh, but it will be so nice to start feeling *normal* again!"

I widened my eyes and tossed my head back, tugging a little at my wig to make sure it covered my bare sideburns.

"Oh, stop. You look beautiful. Just like always." Then she laughed a little. "You know I thought of you when it took me an *hour* to get my hair dry today." Her bright green eyes danced with mischief. "I was pulling it and getting mad, argh!" She dragged her arms away from her hair imitating her arduous beauty regime. "And then I thought, just for a minute, how nice it is for Aime just to pop her perfect hair with the perfect hairstyle right on her head. Hah!"

I laughed back at her, "You're right. That part is nice. I can take two or three showers a day because it's so much faster to get ready! And you know," I lowered my voice and leaned in, "I'm getting a little hair back!"

"Yeah?" She nodded, encouraging me to go on.

"It's almost..." I hesitated, thinking of a comparison, and remembering her husband's generously receding, let's just say balding, hairline, "...it's not quite as much as Chris has."

She snorted and put her arm around my shoulders.

"Hey. It's progress. And in the meantime, you keep rocking those eyelashes!"

Week Fourteen

I breezed into the Women's Cancer Center feeling great. The sky was a deep blue, and a breeze kept the sun from feeling too hot. The air had a crisp quality, so if I had been in Boston it would have felt like fall was around the corner. But in Northern California it was a banner late June day, and I was beginning to enjoy the slower pace of the summer life in the country with the kids. My body was used to the Taxol by then, and I felt somewhat normal, comparatively speaking, of course. That day I was due for round six of twelve, so I was really on the downhill cruise.

I was thrilled that I was starting to grow back some hair. Every day I sat on the counter between the double sinks in our bathroom and peered into the mirror at the little sprouts of hair budding from my head. I couldn't say it was thick, but it was definitely hair—new hair—all growing at the same time. I could make out a faint hair line.

My brisk pace matched my mood as I imagined hair growing under my wig even as I walked. My oversized sunglasses covered the false eyelashes and penciled-in brows. My skin had started to lose the withered yellow tinge that had been a symptom of the AC, and while still pale, I was gaining a tiny bit of color back. If someone didn't look too closely, I was the picture of health. Even Catherine had assured me that with my sunglasses and wig on, I looked "really normal."

Which is why minutes later as I looked into the sympathetic but guarded eyes of the oncologist nurse, my good mood was dashed in an instant.

"Your white blood cell count took a pretty big drop this week, so we're going to have to talk about the booster shots again," she said somewhat cautiously, pointing toward the columns of numbers and abbreviations on her computer screen as if she needed backup proof.

She did need backup. I was incredulous.

"What? I feel fine. I can't do the shots again. That's going to really throw me back. I can't do those shots again," I said, waving my hands in protest.

"The shots we give during Taxol are different from the ones you got during your rounds of AC. We can't let you continue treatment with counts this low. It could be very dangerous. I know you have young children, and we're heading into the Fourth of July weekend where you might be around crowds of people. Our only options are for you to either take the shots or delay treatment for a week and hope that your counts go back up on their own." She stood back from me and crossed her arms, carefully scanning the expression on my face while waiting for me to decide.

It was clever of her to put it that way. Giving me the choice, when really I was having to choose between two options that really stunk. She had said it in a casual voice like a waiter asking, "Soup or salad?" but what I heard was, "Do you want me to cut off your index finger or your pinky?"

"What was your main side effect with the Nulasta shot during AC?" she asked.

"The bone pain," I said, remembering. Bone pain didn't begin to describe the horrible shooting pain that jumped from sternum to rib cage to knees to ankle joints to hip joints like some hammer-wielding maniac hovering over my body, waiting for me to feel some relief before he took the next swing.

"Well, the effects of the Nulasta were probably compounded from the AC, but I can give you Vicodin to see if that helps."

Great, I thought. Just dope me up. We were layering chemicals upon chemicals, trying vainly to find a concoction that worked and hoping the strain wouldn't burn out my liver.

"I guess I don't really have a choice." I sighed, blinking the tears back.

"You always have a choice. You are in the driver's seat," she insisted, with that phrase they must have been coached to say like a politician's talking points.

"I have to keep moving forward. I need to get this over with. So no, I don't have a choice. Any delay is just ripping more weeks away from my life." And no, I thought to myself. I am not in the driver's seat. If I had been driving this whole time, I would not have pulled into the cancer park.

"So let's move on then," she said as she motioned me back onto the table to perform my hundredth breast exam.

At that moment, an administrator knocked on the door announcing Shelley's presence as she waltzed into the room bearing my favorite green tea lemonade. She had her typical bright and beautiful smile and was, as always, perfectly put together and polished with her crisp white Armani jacket, dark skinny jeans and Manolo slides. She plopped her bag down on the chair next to the examining table and looked at me, her smile turning into a puzzled look as she read the expression on my face and saw evidence of recent tears.

"What's going on?"

I filled her in on the update, careful to be as clinical as possible to get the details out without tearing up again.

"Okay," she said, cautiously looking between the nurse and me. "So let me be sure I understand. These shots you have taken before have been really uncomfortable, but you have to take them in order to keep going with the treatments."

I nodded.

"Okay. You can do this. It's just one more thing, and now we're one step closer to the goal. Just think. One step closer to our biggest problem being chipped toenail polish. We do, of course, have to keep the ultimate goal in mind. I'm not hanging out with you at Stanford forever." She tossed her hair back flippantly in order to most advantageously show her blonde locks.

Finally, I cracked a smile and laughed. The nurse took advantage of my lighter mood to finish up quickly. I dressed, and Shelley and I strolled out of the office and up to the infusion center together.

"Hey, at least you got some Vicodin out of it," Shelley said. "I will need to borrow some for my next bikini wax."

I laughed and said, "Yeah, really."

"No, I'm serious," she said. "It's the only way I can do it. One before and one after!"

I pulled into the driveway of the cottage after another trip to Stanford for my booster shot the next day and saw the trucks from the tree service gathered in the burned-out summer grass. They had been doing a lot of work on the trees throughout the property over the past couple of months—trimming the dead branches and keeping them healthy. There was an outbreak of sudden oak death that they had also been careful to watch for, and they marked sick trees with a red plastic tie with the intention of taking the tree down once permission was granted from the town.

I saw a couple of grand old trees along the drive with new red ribbons around them, and my heart sank. It seemed that the disease had spread farther than they thought.

I opened the front door and dropped my bag and keys on the antique mahogany chest next to the entry. My gaze automatically shifted to the glass doors across the room that led out to the patio where my chair beckoned me under the great old oak. I crossed the room, pulled open the door and saw it.

There was a red tie around the tree. My tree. The tree that I sat under every day, letting my mind drift as I watched the squirrels and birds hop and flit among its branches. In my weakened state I had come to think of the tree as a loving grandmotherly figure silently standing by me while I tried to hold onto my strength. And now that strong steadfast tree had shown disease of her own.

Oh, no, no, no, no, no, I thought, pushing my way through the heavy sliding glass doors and out to the tree. I reached both hands out and touched the rough bark tenderly, letting my forehead rest against her trunk. My eyes welled up and the tears spilled over.

I'm so sorry, I whispered to her. I didn't know you were sick too.

The kids were devastated when they saw the red ribbon around the tree after school. We made a family decision to cut the ribbon down and hold it with a rock on the other side of the tree, so the tree guys would still see it, but we wouldn't have to look at it every day. We knew the process of obtaining permission for tree removal could take some time and hoped it would not be soon.

I struggled to get through that round and started relying more heavily on the Ativan and Vicodin. Every afternoon the pain kicked up, and I had to take a Vicodin. I compared the pain to what I had felt once when I had a broken foot. The break began with a sharp, wincing pain, then a dull throbbing pain that came and went with pressure until it finally subsided. The bone pain from the booster shot was a much deeper and more intense pressure that felt as if my bones were crumbling from the inside. The pain would last about fifteen minutes in one spot—in one large bone, such as my sternum or my femur—then move to another like my hips. I would lie in my bed, staring up at the beamed ceiling, waiting for the fifteen minutes to pass before the Vicodin brought the initial wave of relief. The next hour would be spent in a whimpering haze until I could rouse myself to say goodnight to the kids. Then I took an Ativan so that I could sleep through it. Every night that would happen. I fought it at first, waiting to take them until I was desperate, but after a while it became routine. I reasoned to myself that if drugs had gotten me into the mess, the least they could do was help me deal with it. The team and I all agreed that at that point, I should do whatever it took to get to the end.

CHAPTER 21

Other People's Problems

July—Week Sixteen

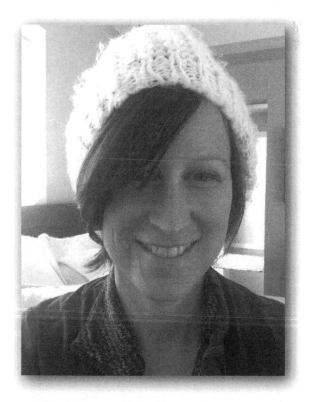

THEN MY LIFE and chemo continued. I didn't want to have a dirty car and a messy house and clothes that didn't fit, but all of those things took time and energy to take care of, neither of which I had. My planters slowly died from neglect. I'd like to say they didn't survive the move, but really I couldn't figure out how to get the water to drain properly, and fixing it never became a priority, so I had to watch the leaves turn yellow and fall off while I spent more and more hours planted under the tree.

When people asked me how I was, then talked to me about being stressed about managing their maintenance appointments like going to the gym, waxing, haircuts and mani-pedis, summer camp, and choir practice, I'm sorry—it seems horribly mean—but I hated them a little bit for it. I hated them for being so shallow and selfish and what I used to be. There were pieces of who I was wrapped up in their words, and they sickened me. I hated them for needing to talk to me about it. Because if they couldn't help me, or at least be positive, I just wanted them to leave me alone. I didn't have a single second to spend on them or their imaginary problems. I guess they didn't realize that while they were scheduling their hair blowouts, I was wondering after each blood test if the doctor would call me and tell me that my cancer had spread, that there was no point in continuing treatment, that I was dying. While they were bitching about the $600 basketball coach, I was worrying about my children, not about carting them all around but just making sure they knew how much I loved them. Every day when I told them I loved them I silently prayed that the words would travel deep inside their souls so that if I ever had to leave them they would always feel the part of me I left behind. That is what I was thinking about if I seemed a little distracted.

As the Taxol continued to build in my system, it became harder and harder to manage. Just when I was beginning to enjoy some semblance of normalcy for a few weeks, I was right back into the thick of things, and it was wearing me down. I stared at my fingernails coming away from the quicks at the tips and reflected on my hair loss, weight loss, loss of elasticity in my skin, loss of shine in my eyes—all the things that were the outward evidence of my cells dying. I wondered what else must be happening to my organs and tissues on the inside. The irony was that I felt at my best on the day of the infusion. I didn't know if it made it easier to keep going, or worse.

So for the eighth round of Taxol, I sat in the waiting room of the infusion center again, Shelley keeping me company after we shared a big Italian lunch at Carpaccio's. The nurse called my name and we were led back into the treatment rooms. Shelley made a point of looking away while I weighed in. After I teased her about it, she said, "Well, that's even more personal than a breast exam."

"It's in kilograms, anyway, so unless you know the conversion rate offhand, I think I'm safe," I retorted.

"In that case you would be right, but I can find out anything on my phone." She winked.

The nurse patiently worked to set me up while Shelley fussed that I was placed in the middle of the room instead of at my favored window seat. She shifted around uncomfortably in the chair next to my reclined infusion Lazy Boy.

"Don't you want a private room? It seems so noisy today."

"I'd rather have the natural light. Those fluorescent bulbs start to get to me after a while."

"I know. They really could use some redecorating in here." A harpist had started up next to us, but the room was so noisy and crowded, it faded into the background. "The harp can stay, but we really need to do something about the color on the walls, and the lighting."

"I agree, and the linoleum on the floor sort of bums me out," I said.

Shelley turned to me then and said, "Scott's not coming today?"

I shook my head. "He's been really bogged down with work lately. All the time he's had to take off for me and to help with the kids has set him back a little. Plus, I think he feels like if you're here, he's got me covered. He really appreciates how much you've helped. You know we both do."

I smiled at Shelley but inwardly cringed at the implied criticism of Scott. I felt protective of him, and it always upset me when people didn't understand him. I hoped that Shelley of all people would. He was quiet, he was calm and steady, and some people might have thought he was aloof, but that wasn't who he was at all. He had been so relieved at my choice of our wedding song because that told him that I knew where his heart was. It was an old country song that had most recently been sung by Alison Krauss called, "When you say nothing at all." The lyrics explained my sentiments exactly: "The smile on your face lets me know that you need me/ There's a truth in your eyes saying you'll never leave me/ A touch of your hand says you'll catch me if ever I fall/ You say it best when you say nothing at all."

My ringing phone interrupted my thoughts, and I dug through my purse to see who it was. I had to fish around all the things I had stuffed in my bag for the day because I had long since given up packing the recommended chemo survival kit in favor of shoving a couple of snacks and a magazine with a sweater and some mints into whatever purse I had been carrying last.

I finally found my phone and checked the screen. It was my brother, Rob. "Hey, Rob, how's it going?"

"Hey, Aime. Just checking in to see how you're doing. We've been thinking about you."

"I'm doing pretty well. At the hospital. It's a chemo day, so you know how those go."

"Oh, right now?" He let out a nervous laugh. "I'm sorry, you don't have to talk."

"No, it's fine. Today is probably one of the better ones, you know? How's Fronda doing?"

"She's doing as well as can be expected. It's tough."

"Tell me about it." We spent a few minutes comparing notes before we said our good-byes. Fronda was in the midst of her heavy treatment and, as expected, it was hitting her hard, but she was getting through it.

I hung up the phone and looked at Shelley, who had been flipping through a magazine.

"My brother," I said.

She raised her eyebrow. "And he wanted to talk about Fronda's health to you, today?"

"Oh, it's fine. I answered the phone, and I asked him about it."

"Well." She huffed a little, then let it go.

Just as I was starting to settle in, I felt a quickening under my rib cage. I had felt the sensation before but only in my back, and it had been fleeting. The sensation fluttered and pulsed a few more times, and I shifted in my seat. I started to pull away from the conversation as my body began to feel lighter. I fussed around in my purse trying to ground myself while I muttered, "Something's wrong. I'm not feeling great." My vision blurred a little, and I blurted, "I think I might pass out."

Shelley watched me carefully while I reached over and pushed the call button and we waited. "I think I'm okay. It's just something feels weird." I felt clammy, my vision was dotted at the edges and I felt myself start to float over my body.

Before I knew it, I was fully reclined and four nurses were surrounding me asking questions. I needed to make the call about whether we could keep going with the infusion. Whenever delay was mentioned, I seemed to tap into some inner strength because I would not, could not, delay. I had to get this over with, despite all my fears.

The floating feeling slowly subsided, and I gritted my teeth.

"No, I have to keep going. Just stay with me," I said to the nurse.

"Okay, we'll start it slow and see how it goes," she said.

"I have to keep going, for God's sake, I just have to do this four more times!" I was shaking with frustration and my eyes brimmed with tears. My anger seemed to give me the extra boost of adrenaline that I needed, and I forced my body to calm down.

Shelley grabbed my hand, her eyes tearing. "We will get you through this. You're going to get through." She looked away and wiped her eyes.

A couple of the nurses cried with us, and we carried on.

On the way out to the car, Shelley turned to me. "Hey," she said, "at least your lashes stayed on."

When I got home, the babysitter Judy had the kids fed, entertained, and ready for bed. It was such a comfort coming home to the evening rituals in progress. Judy had stepped in like a family member, calm and sweet, and the house was always as neat as a pin. I was so glad we had found her. There were some things that had gone my way after all.

I checked in on the kids, inhaling their sweet scents as I kissed each of their heads. Judy gave me a concerned look, asking if I was okay. I nodded and asked her to stay just a while longer until Scott got home so I could lie down. I went into my room, closed the door, and fell to sleep as soon as my body was horizontal.

Then I experienced one of the most insidious side effects of chemotherapy. The nightmare.

Since Mom had died she'd visited me many times in my dreams. Other dreams of her had been of sharing love. Once I saw her waving to me on a crowded street, calling to me that she loved me. Another time I couldn't remember the words we had said, but I woke with warm, happy feelings after sharing a seemingly endless and deeply satisfying conversation about life with her.

On that night, however, we stood alone in a dark room while she floated just above me, draped in white antique laces and gauzy silks. She looked young and beautiful as she always did in my dreams, her dark hair shiny and long and her face full of color and life. She smiled lovingly to me as she motioned to me with her arms and called, "Aime, come with me. Come with me.... Aime.... It's all right.... You can be with me.... Come with me."

I stared at her, enchanted, mesmerized by her movements and her voice until what she was asking dawned on me. "No!" I screamed and pushed at her while she clung to me. "It's not my time. It's not my time!"

I woke panting and fighting against the sheets that seconds earlier had been her arms. It was a hideous trick of the brain, a calling card from all the toxicity. As if what it was doing to my body were not enough, the chemo clawed insidiously into my subconscious, infecting even my cherished connection to my mother and forcing me to push her away.

Scott's steady breathing calmed me, and I was finally able to coax myself back into a deep, dreamless sleep.

Everyone in the family had called me by the next day, somehow sensing my inner struggle. Even Pluto started hunting for me, catching two big field mice and leaving them on the outdoor rug in the middle of the gathering of chairs on the patio. Maverick camped out by my door, and I woke in the night with Scott's arm wrapped protectively over my shoulders.

Recovering from that round was tough, and I camped out in my room again. I had gotten into the habit of taking selfies. The process had started out more optimistically as a way to journal my way through the process, then seemed to take a darker, more desperate turn as if I were a prisoner scratching my name in the wall: "I wuz here."

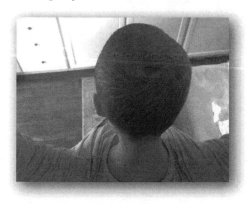

I always had my phone with me to stay on top of emails, and my heart sank when I saw Jennifer's name in my email. She was another mom whose daughter was in Catherine's class at Episcopal who had recently shared with me that she had also been diagnosed with breast cancer. I knew she was having her surgery soon, and I wanted to hear her news.

Hi Aime,

Looks like my chances of getting chemo are higher than I thought. My research says the statistics for relapse are the most important as relapse tends to be stage IV metastatic cancer with a two year survival.

She ran through a number of dizzying statistics and variables before continuing with her main point.

My chemo regimen would be taxotere and cytoxan. Is that what you got? If so brutal honesty about how you've felt each time would be great. Would you have been able to work? Would you have wanted time off? When do you feel worst, and when do you feel better?
Do you notice changes in cognition?
Also where did you get your gorgeous wig?

Thanks!
Jennifer

My stomach soured. I leaned my head back against the cushions and closed my eyes, massaging my temples and letting out a long, slow breath. I wondered incredulously what lapse of consideration had allowed her to press send on the missive—as if I had ever had the choice of whether or not to do chemo myself.

I breathed slowly while my heart pounded with anger. Scott walked into the room to tell me dinner was ready and raised an eyebrow at my expression.

I unloaded. "Am I being unreasonable?" I asked when I was finished my tirade, wanting him to tell me what I was missing for Jennifer's sake.

"No, you're not," he surprised me by agreeing. "Just ignore her and deal with it when you can." He clearly didn't think the woman's feelings were worth the energy it was taking from me.

I, on the other hand, did not want to turn my back on someone who was just then being faced with one of her life's most difficult situations. She was grasping at straws and reaching out for help from anyone and everyone she could find. I, having had a similar diagnosis and a child of the same age in school, seemed a likely resource for her. What she didn't know was that while she felt like she was drowning, so did I. Just the fact that I was a few months into the process only served to make me more exhausted, and while she grasped at me through the water, I was struggling to stay afloat myself. Any extra weight threatened to pull me under. So I responded to her email and then regretfully pushed her away, hoping she would find stronger resources than me.

Hi Jennifer,

Looks like you are in much better shape than me, that's something! Since my tumor was grade 3 with lymph involvement I am doing a more aggressive form of chemo—so thank your lucky stars because being totally frank it completely sucks and there is no way I could have worked through at least 3-4 separate weeks. My work is the kids and I had to outsource and rely on help for the better part of 4 of 8 weeks not including the surgery and whatever I have to deal with upcoming. Although everyone is different. My sister in law is going through ac now and it's not hitting her as hard—she's 7 yrs older than me and supposedly the younger you are the harder it can hit (some-thing about active cells- I'm 41). Now after round 8/12 of taxol I could work but I would have to miss a lot of time for ap-pointments and infusions. I had cytoxan with adriamycin dose dense followed by taxol. Taxol is not that bad, but now a little more than halfway through the cumulative effect is wearing me down. I think the cytoxan wouldn't have been that bad by itself. You might even use the ice caps and keep your hair. I didn't have a shot at that so they told me not to bother. The cogni-tive issues were definitely worse during the ac rounds—on the worst days I couldn't focus on conversation or even tv more than 30 minutes, but now (and for the last 6 wks at least) I've been reading voraciously and am even back to writing when I feel like it—now it's more getting my head in the right frame as opposed to concentration. I would think a desk job would be ok—you might be operating at 80 percent or so generally.

Sorry if this sounds negative—maybe if you asked me when it's actually done, and for sure yours wouldn't be this bad because it's a different protocol. Just saying—chemo didn't get its bad rep for no reason, it's a Herculean effort of mental, emotional and physical strength to get through by anyone's standards—that being said, looking at the kids there is nothing I wouldn't do to have the chance to hold my grandchildren.
Good luck,
Aime

Between my sister in law, Jennifer, and women I would see all the time at the cancer center, I reached a moment where it all just started to get to me. I didn't want to be in that "club." It wasn't about "why me" or complaining about being sick. I just didn't identify with it. Or rather, I didn't *want* to identify with it. I saw people going bald to the infusion center and wearing sweatshirts with slogans on them to the effect of "beat cancer" as if they were in a sporting event. I was glad for them. I knew it's what got them through it, and God knows, you have to do whatever it takes to get through it. But the thought of wearing a pink ribbon everywhere and tying a sweet little bow on my bald head and going out in public made me want to vomit. I just wanted to put on my wig and my fake eyelashes and throw on my white skinny jeans (two sizes smaller thanks to the chemo diet) with my strappy sandals and walk into the world feeling pretty good on my good days. A stranger might not even be able to tell. It was none of their business, and I didn't want to bum them out having to worry about that nice lady with cancer.

I just couldn't relate to all those "bald and proud" women who seemed to have joined some type of sorority. I guess I've never been good at clubs, and while I could chat with the person sitting next to me in the infusion center about the ins and outs of chemo all day, don't you dare ask me to take my wig off. Nobody needed to see that.

I was sick and tired of being sick and tired and so angry at being pulled at. I can't help you, I thought. I can't even help me. All of my control had slipped through my fingers, and I was left floating free form in the dark void. I just prayed that someone had left me a rope.

CHAPTER 22

The Chemo Song
Week Seventeen

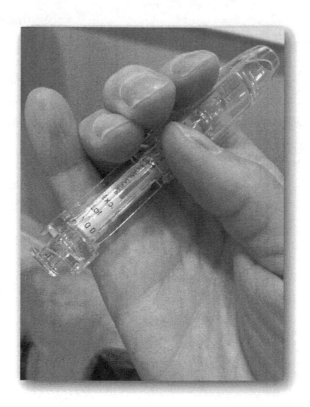

CATHERINE'S BIRTHDAY WAS coming up and I couldn't manage a party, so Scott had cleverly asked her if there were any trips she would like to take instead. She'd been wanting to go to Universal Studios in

Southern California, so we got the okay from the doctors for a few days away and Scott planned the trip. We would take the quick flight to LA, and I could camp out by the hotel pool while Scott took the kids to Universal. Then we would drive up the coast to Santa Barbara, have a couple of relaxing days at the beach, and fly home from there. I think we all agreed that a change of pace and a quick weekend away would do each of us some good.

At my next infusion, the nurse taught Scott how to give me the Neupagen shot, so we could leave the following morning. I watched dubiously as his massive hands grasped the needle and jabbed it into the practice plastic "flesh." He seemed confident, though, and the nurse nodded at him and touched my arm reassuringly.

"He'll do fine," she said.

Scott had been feeling a little boxed out from my chemo days, so I think he was glad to step back in while Shelley was traveling. By that point he had rushed to show up several times only to find the two of us chatting away about a variety of issues he had nothing to add to, so he would pull out his computer to bang out some emails, feeling like his presence was completely unnecessary. I loved for him to be there, but I loved for him to be able to take care of me at home more, so if there were a choice, and if I had other visitors, he was officially off the hook.

After Scott had his injection tutorial, we enjoyed a quiet hour catching up about our plans, hopes and dreams. Scott never hesitated to talk about the future. He never seemed to have the doubt that this would be more than a temporary setback like I did. We reminisced about summers in Boston, our favorite season there. We hoped that one day we could buy a little beach cottage somewhere in Essex or Gloucester because we wanted to have a solid anchor there. He talked about retirement and how he wanted to spend half of his time in Marin and half in Boston, taking the most advantage of both coasts. I dreamed with him, but my dreams were more hesitant. Where his felt like plans, mine felt more like wishes on a star.

Early the next morning we woke for the flight to LA and Scott stuck the needle in my belly like a pro. It seemed to go against a primal survival instinct to expose my belly to someone wielding a sharp object, but he had earned that kind of trust. He didn't even leave a bruise. It was a new milestone in our relationship.

We made our way through the LA traffic out to Santa Monica and found our hotel, and the kids jumped into their swimsuits immediately. Scott took them down to the pool while I napped in the cool air-conditioned room. As much as the travel put an extra strain on me, time in a hotel melted it away. Just knowing that everything we needed was within reach was a huge relief. The four of us were never happier than when we were exploring new places together, and I loved it when we were all crammed into one room. I felt like a mama dog who was content with all her puppies around her.

By dinner I had regained my energy, and we all headed out to the Santa Monica Pier. We walked down the steep slope to the boardwalk, and Scott looked at me and grimaced. "Think you'll be okay getting back up?"

I shrugged. "As long as we take it grandma slow."

The afternoon sun shone down on us while the ocean breeze kissed our faces. The kids both stayed near us, being a little protective of me. We walked into the crowd on the boardwalk, and Catherine and Wesley both lit up at the carnival atmosphere. Music was blaring, and the smell of cotton candy and popcorn was thick in the air.

"Let's play a game!" Catherine shouted, pointing at the ball toss, her gaze fixated on the giant stuffed animals dangling around the booth.

"Rides first!" Wesley jumped up, his eyes widening as he took in the huge roller coaster.

I sat down on one of the benches while Scott chased after the kids for an hour. We found a fish shack for dinner then headed back up the hill, the kids spent but happy.

I struggled a bit with the incline, and Scott put his hand on my back and raised his eyes at me.

"Want a push?" he teased.

"Remember when you had to do that when I was pregnant with Wesley and we were walking up the hill from the Warren Tavern in Charlestown?" I asked him.

"Yes, and I think you might have had him the next day." He chuckled. "He was so big."

"Oh, I know. Nine pounds, three ounces, all solid. He came out looking like he was three months old." Lifted by the happy memories, I was able to make it up the hill. By the time we got back to the hotel, we were all wiped out and crashed in the room.

I planted myself by the hotel pool the next day while they all went to Universal Studios. They had been particularly excited about the new *Despicable Me* exhibit. Catherine was a little worried about leaving me alone, and though I assured her I was fine by the pool with a book, she still checked in throughout the day, sending me pictures and a couple of videos she had taken.

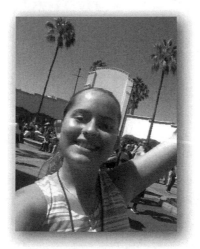

My favorite was a selfie video while she was on a Ferris wheel. She waved to the camera, then put on her serene smile and gazed out over the park before turning the camera around to show the view. Tween budding filmmaker.

The next day we drove up the coast to Santa Barbara, stopping on the way at a trendy lunch spot in Malibu. We stayed at the Fess Parker Double Tree in Santa Barbara, a big family hotel right across from the beach. Shelley texted to see how things were going.

Shelley: Send me pictures of all the good looking guys at the pool.
Aime: Are there supposed to be some? I haven't seen any at the Fess Parker!
Shelley: That's right, what good looking guy hangs out at the Fess Parker???
Aime: I know. That's part of the problem, I think. (wink)
Shelley: Good looking guys don't say, "Hey lets hang at the Fess Parker" It's dads that get a good deal on expedia
Aime: hahahahaha

The temperature in Santa Barbara was perfect, a balmy 82 degrees and sunny. It hardly ever got that warm on the coast of Northern California, especially in the foggy summer months, so we took advantage of every minute and lingered for hours on the beach. I lounged under an umbrella while the kids surfed the waves for hours with Scott bouncing back and forth between us. I didn't want to take my wig off, so I still couldn't swim, but I waded into the ocean up to my waist, much to the excitement of the kids who clung to me like giant starfish.

On the last night we had an early dinner and went back to the room, everyone tired and happy from all the sun and fresh air. We didn't have dessert with dinner and our food had been pretty light, so we all started feeling a little hungry as we watched a movie.

"Oh, let's see if we can get some of those cookies they have when you check in." I said, suddenly craving something sweet.

"Oh, yes. Those are so yummy!" Wesley immediately starting to bounce on the bed in anticipation.

Catherine got out the room service menu and said, "There is also a brownie and ice cream dessert. Hmmm? Can we? Can we, Mom?" She put her face close to mine with the teasing puppy dog eyes she uses when she's begging for something.

I looked at Scott and he opened his eyes wide, then smiled and said, "Sure, if you want to."

"Let's do it!" I ordered room service, and by the time they got there we were all bouncing on the bed in excitement. I had even thrown caution to the wind and left my scarf on instead of changing into my wig when the waiter came in. Other than his quick nervous glance toward my head, it didn't even matter. It was by far the best dessert I had ever had, the brownie and ice cream oozing into each other and melting in my mouth with every bite. I looked into the happy eyes of my children and for a moment felt total bliss.

Week Nineteen

It was another typical bright sunny summer day, and I had left the kids home with Judy while I went to the cancer center. I had long since followed Shelley's lead and given my car to the valet, figuring if ever the twelve dollar expense was worth it, it was then. That day was Taxol Eleven—my fifteenth round of chemotherapy, nineteen weeks in.

I walked through the sliding glass doors, flipping my sunglasses up on my wig as the vents blew the hair out of place and I tucked it back behind my ears. The whole routine had become disgustingly familiar. Blood, needles, poison. Just another day.

Dr. S was happy to report that my blood cell count went back up, so I could skip the booster shot that week. After we high-fived in celebration, I asked why she thought that had happened. She smiled and said, "Seems like a little fun and relaxation with your family was good for you."

Of all the things I was struggling to do and all the advice I was desperately following—from acupuncture to a restrictive diet and a blend of supplements—the thing that seemed to help the most was so simple. Joy. Happiness. Love. These things had literally changed my body chemistry.

The boost lasted about a week, then the dreaded cumulative effects of Taxol started to take over. Most days I would plod along wearily until the late afternoon, then I would plop some dinner on the table and disappear into my room. I lay prone on my bed counting the beams on the ceiling trying to survive the crushing bone pain rotating through my joints and largest bones before I gave into the Vicodin and Ativan haze again. I was ashamed by it, but I was so weak that I would have to ask Catherine to bring me water when she came into my room to visit. Wesley hardly ever came in during those days.

I struggled into the kid's room to put Wesley to bed, sitting down on the reading chair while he brushed his teeth and leaning against the rail of his loft while I breathlessly sang his baby song. I kissed him goodnight, then went straight back to bed. Catherine usually joined me then, and the two of us read in silence, listening to the television Scott had tuned into baseball in the living room. Sometimes I would gaze over at her, simply absorbing and adoring the fact that she was there. She was so steady and sweet and helpful and caring, and it broke my heart that she had to be the strong one at twelve years old.

One week later we all crowded into the exam room together. Scott and Shelley sat in the chairs while I sat on the table with Dr. D, the surgeon, Dr. S, and a couple of RNs standing in front of us. Dr. D said everything felt good, but he ordered a couple of pre-surgical scans in the next couple of weeks before my follow-up surgery to clear the margins and check my lymph nodes again. Dr. S was just happy to see me with passable blood tests at the last infusion appointment, which only meant that my vital organs were functioning to some degree and my blood count, while low, was high enough for one last round. She sensed the celebratory mood in the air, as everyone did. It was finally there, the last day of chemo. The tape at the end of the marathon. I understood why so many people collapsed at the finish line dissolving into a puddle of tears and sweat.

Before we moved on to the infusion center, Dr. S, queen of the understatement, touched my arm, looked at me seriously and said, "I don't want to take anything away from this moment, but you should know—it's going to take some time for you to start feeling like yourself, like Aime, again."

"I know," I said.

"I mean it," she said, seeming not to believe me. "Probably a year. It'll probably be next summer before you start really feeling fully like yourself."

She didn't think it was sinking in, but it was. I believed her.

The next few hours went off flawlessly, with many of the nurses I had gotten to know over the weeks stopping by to say their congratulations. Shelley made sure to ask the nurse about the "chemo song" she had seen sung to others on their last day. I imagined it was the equivalent of someone asking the waiter at the restaurant for the birthday song, and I felt much the same happy embarrassment.

So when I was all done the nurses gathered around singing, "The chemo's done and we're so excited for you, hey ya, hey ya, the chemo's done," to the tune of "My Boyfriend's Back." They all wore sombreros and did a little dance as the lines went on. Then they all cheered and one by one came over to give me hugs. It was a beautiful moment and a happy send-off.

Scott and Shelley both looked on with proud smiles on their faces and Shelley joked, "Those sombreros remind me that Dr. S said she would go for margaritas with us to celebrate! We need to have a party! This is such a momentous occasion. It must be marked appropriately."

Scott raised his eyebrows. "Do you feel like margaritas?"

I laughed, "Maybe not today, but soon. I am certain that at some point I will want a margarita again."

"Well, okay, if you're sure," Shelley said, a little disappointed.

My nurse came over grinning widely. "That was the biggest group for the chemo song I've ever seen."

"Oh really? That's so sweet." I smiled back at her. She'd been my favorite nurse, and I'd had her several times by then. I so appreciated her calm, matter-of-fact demeanor and the way she spoke to me like a friend. She had held my hand and cried for me when I almost had to quit, and she stayed with me every session after that.

"Yeah, I just went out to the nurse's station to let them know, and everyone wanted to come over today. We're all so happy for you!" She took off the port access and disconnected the IV swiftly. "And now you are free to go!"

I hugged her one more time. I knew it must be one of the best parts of her job to send patients home knowing they were finally done.

"Thank you for being such a rock star at your job," I said.

Walking away I looked around to say good-bye to this place for what I hoped was the last time. This place where I had spent so many hours, and such emotion. And while I was so relived to be done, I knew Dr. S was right. It wasn't really over. I still had to manage that day's infusion over the following few days, not to mention the upcoming surgery, six weeks of radiation, and adjusting to hormone therapy. To try to get back to what might feel like myself again would be a slow climb. And honestly, I didn't even know who I was anymore. Whatever or whoever I was climbing toward was not the same person I was before. I hardly remembered who she was.

Five days later we were on a plane to Seattle. The flight was quick and we packed everything we needed for the week in four carry-on bags. We rode in a taxi with the windows down from the airport through

228

downtown Seattle past the Seahawks stadium and the Starbucks headquarters right to the pier where the cruise ship we would take to Alaska was waiting. The embarking process was smooth, and before long we were settling into a sizeable room with a long balcony stretching along the side.

Scott and the kids went immediately to explore the boat and find the best snack spots while I unpacked and fell onto the bed. I looked around the room and out the sliding glass doors and windows. I nodded to myself and closed my eyes. Step one, I thought. Step one toward feeling normal again. A family vacation.

After about an hour, Scott and the kids came back to the room, and the captain announced over the speakers that we would be departing. The kids wanted to swim while we cruised past Seattle, so we all went up to the pool deck and watched the space needle and the Seattle skyline grow smaller and smaller in the distance.

The next few days brought more and more adventures—exploring the cruise ship, spotting pods of whales from the deck, sailing through a fjord to view a glacier from the ship, and stopping along the way in little coastal Alaskan towns, some of which are only accessible by boat or plane. We saw huge lazy humpbacks lounging with full bellies in clear still water between the little islands off the coast and ate tons of salmon.

One of our favorite stops was Sitka, where we went to a raptor center that rehabilitated injured or orphaned bald eagles and a bear fortress that saved grizzly bear cubs. The bears were kept in a defunct water treatment plant with giant circular stone structures acting as their enclosures. They were in their natural environment with ponds to swim in and trees to climb on but according to Alaska law would never be able to be released back into the wild. The bear "cubs" were massive animals with deep thick brown fur and claws that must have been five or six inches long. The man who ran the fortress carried a bucket of salmon heads that he tossed to the bears. One female bear came over asking for more salmon and calmly scratched her claws along the side of her enclosure like a cat scratching the side of a post, creating a sound like knives on cement that echoed up to us while we watched a mere ten feet away from the overhang. She made a muffled growling sound and was rewarded with a fish head tossed her way, which she promptly caught in her mouth before giving a grunt of thanks and ambling away.

After spending a lot of time watching the bears, we walked through the town park in Sitka, which was home to multiple totem poles and several streams. The streams were filled with salmon, thousands of them, each at least two feet long swimming side by side and easily visible through the crystal clear water. As we walked back toward the pier where our ship was docked, we caught sight of a bald eagle flying overhead. We stopped at a little restaurant and ordered salmon sandwiches, which turned out to be filled with the freshest, most flavorful and perfectly cooked salmon we had ever tasted.

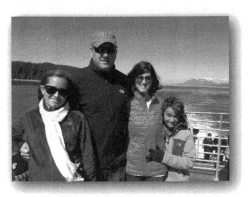

Every day my energy improved, and I felt a little better than the day before. The next day we had our big excursion in Ketchikan, where we went on a floatplane to view the glaciers. None of us had ever been on a float plane before, so the kids were bouncing around with nervous excitement while we waited for our appointed time on a dock with the planes gliding in to land and motoring off in a steady stream.

"What color will our plane be?" Wesley asked.

"I hope it's a red one," Catherine said. "Yellow would be my second choice."

After a few minutes our name was called, our instructions were given, and we were paired with a young man and his daughter and introduced to our captain, Brent, who stood in front of a red plane tied to the dock.

"Is everyone ready to go?" Brent asked once we were all settled in. "It's a spectacularly clear day, so I'm going to head up a little higher than usual. You're going to get a fantastic view of the glaciers. We'll have a little time to stop up there and then we'll head back down. Okay?"

We all gave him the thumbs up, and what felt like a boat turned into a plane as we picked up speed and slowly lifted off up into the air. We flew past the small buildings and boats along the water, and Wesley grabbed my arm and pointed at our cruise ship out the window. The town grew smaller and the plane turned toward the mountains as we began a steady climb in altitude.

Eventually we rose above the mountains, which extended beyond for miles and miles as far as we could see. It was a true glimpse of the vast wilderness that was Alaska. We flew over the white and blue icy glaciers for a few minutes, and the pilot pointed out a glacier lake below us, wedged between a few mountain peaks.

"I'll put the plane down there for a little bit, okay?"

We all nodded enthusiastically, and the plane began to descend. As we got closer and closer to the water between the mountaintops, the little girl on the plane with us started to scream. I looked carefully at Catherine and Wesley to make sure they were all right with this, and they both grinned at me and gave me the thumbs up.

The landing was as smooth as the glassy water and Brent, the pilot, opened up the door to let us walk out onto the pontoons that held the plane afloat. The little girl with her father had calmed down but had no interest in leaving the plane, so the four of us and Brent walked out on the pontoons and squatted down, touching the pure water and soaking in the pristine air. It felt as if we were the only people on the planet.

Eventually Brent said we had to go back, and we reluctantly climbed back into the plane and made our way back down to the coast. I could have sat on the pontoon dangling my feet in the water for hours.

We got back to the cruise ship and the kids decided to go to movie night at the kids club while Scott and I chose one of the dressier restaurants for dinner. Finally we had time to reconnect, just the two of us, relaxed and happy and together.

The rest of the week passed in a fun adventure mode, and I gradually regained my strength along with about four pounds. Catherine and I sat together on the plane back to San Francisco and talked about how the week had gone.

She said, "Just so you know. I don't like the stereotype that teenagers don't like their parents. It's not true."

"I know." I smiled and kissed her forehead. My heart melted and broke into a million pieces at her feet as it had done so many times. I felt like Sally Field accepting the Oscar. *You like me, you really like me*, I thought, but I had known it all along.

CHAPTER 23

Rads
September

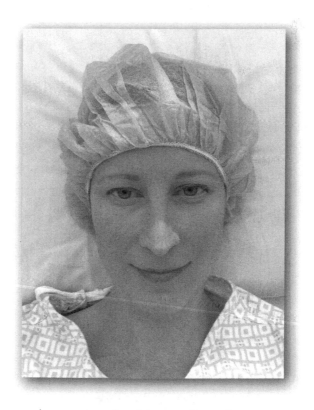

WHEN WE RETURNED home, we had just a few days to get ready for school again, and after settling Catherine into her new school in Woodside and getting Wesley ready for the bump up to third grade back at Episcopal, I was exhausted yet oddly refreshed. I was ready for what I envisioned would be the last great push before this was done.

Catherine started the day before Wesley, so I was able to spend time with each of them making sure they were ready for the year to begin. Catherine's transition to her new school went incredibly smoothly. The school seemed like a sweet, safe environment where there were a lot of opportunities in a relaxed atmosphere. It made me wonder more than passingly why we hadn't been there the whole time.

Wesley ran in to join his friends the next day with such excitement that he barely even turned around to wave good-bye to me. His face lit up with a happy grin under his permanently wild brown hair and I relaxed. They were both settled.

It had been a nice break until yesterday, but it was only the second day of school, and I was thrust right back into it. I lay back against the cushioned exam table, left arm raised high above my head and body positioned slightly on the side to give the ultrasound technician the best view of my armpit as she patiently searched for lymph nodes. It was my last pre-surgery scan, and I was a little anxious about what she might find.

I chatted with the technician. She had been on medical leave during my previous couple of appointments, so we hadn't met before, but she remembered seeing my scans, and she was familiar with my case history. We talked about the summer and about Nashville, my hometown, where she loved to visit. All the while she was moving the scope around under my arm and on the side of my chest, measuring and capturing images on the screen. After a long and thorough exam, she started to wipe the gel away from my skin and I sat up a little.

"Will the radiologist be able to tell me what they see today?" I asked.

"I'm going to go talk to him now, and I'll ask him to come in. Just stay put for a minute, okay?" She nodded at me and went out, pulling the curtain and the door closed behind her.

I shuddered when I thought of the PT scan the day before. I had cried in front of the nurse when she missed my port and had to poke me twice, and I still hadn't heard the results. I thought I was out of the woods with the end of chemo, but I wasn't quite. After a few minutes of staring at the ceiling, I sat up as the radiologist and the technician came back into the room. The radiologist was someone I had never met.

"I wanted to come in and speak with you," he said, looking me directly in the eye while holding up my chart. "I've looked at your ultrasound pictures. We were able to see several of your lymph nodes and they all appear normal."

"Oh, good," I said, exhaling a breath I hadn't been aware I was holding.

"And I saw your PT scan from yesterday and you are totally clear. It showed nothing, absolutely nothing from the base of your skull to your pelvis." He said it in a way that seemed even to surprise him a little.

"Oh. That's good. That's really good." I said, my own smile broadening in return.

The technician nodded behind him, her eyes shining with tears.

"So good luck with the rest of your journey and all the best to you," the doctor said as he left the room. The technician gave my arm a little squeeze before she left. They must have loved giving good news.

I waited for my car from the valet and sent out a quick blast on CareZone. "Great news today! Pre-surgical scans were ALL CLEAR! They will do more tests tomorrow after the surgery, so not totally out of the woods yet, but this is very good news!"

For the rest of the afternoon my phone lit up with congratulations and well wishes for the following day, lifting me up even higher.

Then back in the surgery pre-op room I sat, prepped, waiting again for the team to get started. Looking at Scott next to me, I was thrown suddenly back to the moment when I first knew it would be love. The crisp fall air whipped through my hair as I blasted the plaintive wails of Dave Matthews on the stereo from the mix tape he had sent me. I had spent every last dollar I had on the red convertible that sped over the Tennessee hills, and I knew I would let it all go willingly as I listened over and over to lyrics describing the upside down, tumbled-around feeling of this instant crush.

What no one saw when he missed chemo days and doctor appointments for important meetings was all the nights and weekends. Chemo happened in one day. It was a normal day, one on which I generally felt pretty good. It's what happened after that brought me down to an animal level. I watched countless times the sun fade into the afternoon through the open doors of my bedroom, where from my position prone on the bed I could see him grill up some dinner for the kids, then sit at the patio table, tucking into some heavy meat and a beer while I couldn't even muster the energy to walk the twenty yards between us. He spent all those days and nights alone with the kids while they tried to go on with life around me, my presence lurking in the bedroom never far from their minds. Yet still he whispered to me as he took off my sleeping cap that he didn't care about my hair. He loved me. He just wanted me to be well. He would do anything, he said over and over.

He let me stay in my cave as long as I needed to. He got me mashed potatoes time after time from behind the counter at Roberts Market without ever blinking an eye or suggesting a green salad. He never brought his own agenda to the table. He would put his head down, get his work done, and check in with me. It was the way it had always been, and it was what I loved about him even before I fully understood it. He had always given me the space I needed, and I learned to do the same for him. He needed to see live music every couple of months, ski ten days a year, and get close to the ocean a few times every summer. He was a simple man.

The only other people who glimpsed the reality of the situation were the healthcare workers. I had shielded my friends from the worst parts, but the health team knew, and Scott knew. So many times they had seen a partner leave when the going got rough. They understood that at our age, the prime working years of Scott's career, one that typically had him working sixty- and seventy-hour weeks, the primary caregiver carries a particularly heavy load.

So when he looked at me and laughed at a joke we shared, listened to my endless questions about the minute growth rate of my hair, and snuggled in bed after a long day rubbing my baby hair and agreeing, yes, it's definitely growing, I knew who we were together and would always be.

I got through the surgery well and went back into my cave for the next couple of days to heal. One afternoon I shuffled out to the living room in time for the kids to get home from school. Shelley was dropping them off, and I had tried to make myself presentable, putting on my wig and a nicer wrap around my sweatpants in case she wanted to say hello.

Her car pulled halfway up the drive and then stopped. I saw Maverick sitting calmly in the driveway in front of her car. The windows rolled down and she poked her head out calling to him, then the kids waved and called his name, and he slowly turned his head to the side but remained there. The kids jumped out of the car, waving their good-byes and ran toward the house, ruffling Maverick's fur and calling him a silly dog as they went by. I waved from the door as she backed her car back down the drive. Maverick knew. I needed another day or two in my cave, and he was looking out for me.

The next day I got the results of the pathology report. All clear.

October

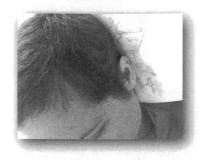

My face pinched up like an angry bird and sparks seemed to flash out of my brightening green and red eyes. My mouth opened and huffed out an almost visible black smoke. The ugly black Sharpie X on my chest bore the brunt of my frustration. As if I hadn't suffered enough indignity. I gave up months of my life in the name of eradicating every last cell of cancer, simply going on the word of the professionals, the highest in their field, the barbarians of the day. I did what they asked me to, and then at the end of it they marked me up with Sharpies and stickers and asked me to leave them for ten days while they made a plan for frying more of my cells...just in case.

It wasn't just the Sharpie that set me off as I ripped off the plastic sticker and saw the ink had seeped deeply below it. It was the size of the X. They hadn't even bothered to be discreet. It wasn't low beneath my breasts; it was high, toward the top of a hint of cleavage, clearly visible under a button-down shirt and easily three times the size of a quarter. They casually marked me up and sent me on my way as if there weren't a chance that I would care to live a life in which Sharpie scrawled over my body was a bother. A birthday dinner for my son, a T-shirt for a ball game, a nightgown worn to make me feel like a woman—I couldn't do any of those things without the ugly sprawling X on my chest.

I had spent the better part of the afternoon getting set up for the next thirty rounds of radiation. It took a team of physicists, doctors, and technicians a week to take my measurements and devise a precise map for the x-rays to hit the targeted areas while leaving my heart, lungs, and other vital organs untouched. The team placed me in a scan machine in the exact location I needed to stay while they created a mold of my back, shoulders, and neck that would be placed under the x-ray every day to keep me in the correct position.

Another team then marked my body with the sharpie Xs and two permanent tattoos, creating a map they would follow for the following weeks. I had lived over forty years without getting a tattoo, and there in the cancer center I got two little blue dots, one on the side of my breast near the scar from my surgery and the other on the rise of my breast over my heart. The last one might be visible when I wore a swimsuit, but it was subtle enough to be a freckle. I might be the only person who saw it easily and clearly every time I looked down at my bare breasts.

When I asked them about all the marks, they said they needed landmarks. I stared at the tiny dot next to my huge scar wondering why that hadn't been enough.

I was facing the next step, six weeks of radiation therapy five days a week (of course they recommended six instead of the normal five because they wanted me to have a "booster"), and I knew my head wasn't in the right place. I just couldn't get it there. I was done with all of it, but it wasn't done with me.

Somewhere in the middle of radiation, Shelley brought Abby over in the afternoon for a playdate and so we could catch up. With the busy fall schedule for the kids and the tax daily radiation appointments were taking on my own schedule, we hadn't been able to sit down and talk for a while. The kids had planned out a specific task to accomplish on

Minecraft, so we left them huddled around the computer while we stretched out on the patio chairs under the old water oaks. I giggled a little at my bare feet next to Shelley's black kitten heels. My own flip-flops had been immediately kicked off and were underneath the ottoman.

We sipped on some iced tea and Shelley sighed and said, "I'm so glad the cottage worked out for you. It's so beautiful here."

"I'm so glad too," I said, listening to the wide variety of birds chirping all around us as we were surrounded by green trees and blue sky. "It's really been perfect."

"I know, if it only had a third bedroom, I'd have locked you into a two-year lease." She shook her head. "I know it's not a permanent solution, but we'll find the next thing when the time is right."

"That's right," I said. "We have some time to think about what the next step will be."

"Have you talked to Lauren lately?" Shelley asked.

I paused, remembering the troubling conversation I had had the day before with Lauren. The two of them had become a little distant in the past few weeks and Shelley seemed hurt. She had talked to me about it, and while I sympathized, I really didn't want to get in the middle of what was turning into a full-blown grown-up girl drama.

Lauren and I had reconnected over the weekend when Scott and her husband planned a family outing. I was glad to be able to move forward with her so that we could remain friends as our husbands had done. While we were catching up Lauren had mentioned sweetly in an "I'm just concerned about her," tone of voice that she thought Shelley should spend less time criticizing other people's husbands and more time focusing on her own marriage.

I was stunned by the loaded statement and defended Shelley, saying I thought they were doing fine, but later I stewed over the words. She must have been talking about Scott, I thought. What other husband would Shelley be criticizing to Lauren?

"I have. I'm sorry that you two are having trouble. It seems like the two of you need a talk-it-out," I said. I wasn't ready to get into my suspicions at the time, but they were bothering me nonetheless, and I was equally eager to avoid the she-said/she-said between two friends.

So Shelley changed the subject. "So how is everything going with you? How is radiation?"

"It's okay," I paused, and she waited. I was growing weary of always having to put a smile on things and pretend that I was able to handle it all. So I decided to be candid. "Actually, I'm pretty tired. People think it's all over, but it's really not. I'm still trying to climb back to normal from chemo, my energy is not even close to where it was, and I have to go back to the cancer center every single day."

Shelley seemed taken aback. "Oh wow." She swallowed and looked at me, staying still. So I continued.

"It's just that everything has changed. I feel like a completely different person. I am overwhelmed just trying to process everything that has happened. My life as I knew it was wiped out, and when I rebuild it I don't want to bring anything negative back in. I have the opportunity here to start fresh, and I am not going to allow myself to get sucked back into things I don't want to be a part of or have in my life." My voice had risen over the last few words so I took a deep breath and looked back up into the trees, feeling the light breeze ruffle my skirt and letting it calm me.

"Wow," Shelley said again. "I had no idea you were going through all of this. Work and school have been so busy, and I've been so distracted and sad about Lauren that I haven't even thought about it. You worked so hard to get through the hardest part, and I just thought it was all over."

"I know." I pulled down my sunglasses against the glare. "I think we all did. But it isn't. It's not going to be over for a while now. In some ways it might not ever be over."

Shelley's eyes welled up with tears, and she looked at me. "I am so sorry. I am still here for you, and you will get through this stage too."

"I know." I smiled at her. "Thanks for letting me vent."

"I'm just glad I know what's going on now. And you can always vent with me."

We said our good-byes, and as I put away the glasses from our tea and tidied up the kitchen, I let the conversations drift back over me.

I hadn't thought too much about it before because I was grateful for the distraction and fun that Shelley provided in a decidedly un-fun environment. But by then I was beginning to understand Shelley's motivations, what was in it for her, why she had wanted to spend all that time hanging out with me in the cancer center. She could feel good about herself, knowing she was helping a friend. And at the end of the day she could go home, and whatever she was dealing with there, she could say, "At least I don't have cancer."

As for the stuff with Lauren- from a distance it looked like high school drama, hurt feelings, game playing, talking behind others' backs, and I frankly didn't have the energy to wade through it all. But at the same time I was grateful for what kind of friend Shelley had been. I supposed I was learning to take the good with the bad and to create boundaries.

But there was something to be said for history, for places and people I had known for more than a decade. It takes time for things to truly become a part of a person's life, time I hadn't had in California. I was just visiting there, and I was having trouble understanding the native language. Some kind souls had been so generous to me when they saw me suffering, but I thought deep down that I didn't belong there. It was not my home. I was like that bird from the children's book asking, "Are you my mother?" It was such a relief for the little bird to finally find his mother in the end. I had lost my mother, but I still had my family, and I could find my way home.

Midway through radiation I had to spend some more time in a scan machine while technicians made a plan for the final "bonus" week of radiation in which they concentrated the x-rays to the highly targeted area of the site where tissue had been removed.

"It reduces your rate of recurrence by 6 percent," my radiation oncologist had assured me.

"Let's do it, then." I had said. All of these raised statistics from additional treatments added up to way more than 100 percent, or I supposed they were fractional increases from smaller and smaller pieces of the pie, but I couldn't begin to sort it all out, so I just did what they told me.

The room was dark and quiet, the only sounds being the hum and occasional soft beeping from the vast array of ultra-high-tech equipment. I lay prone on a flat surface that slid out from the mouth of the great circle that was the scan machine. I had been pushed back and forth through the screen several times, and now the team was using an ultrasound to do the fine-tuning.

My anger at not being done had dissipated, and I was numb again, letting them do whatever it took to get me finished.

"Thar she blows," the technician said in a hushed and slightly awed tone.

A silence hung over the room as we all stared at the ultrasound screen. She had warned me that it might take her some time to map out the cavity that was the hole in my left breast. She was being careful with me because the skin around my breast was a deep and angry red from weeks of radiation, and she knew how sensitive it was.

However, she had barely touched my skin with the probe over my surgery site when the black and white lines of my healthy dense tissue seemed to disappear into a great black cavern. The three of us watched her explore the parameters of this void in my breast looming large on the screen as if we were in a deep-sea submarine charting a great abyss in the ocean. That familiar sense of vertigo overcame me again, and it was hard to know which end was up.

It took both technicians less than an hour to map what they called the cavity, the large hole in my breast the size of a plum that was currently filled with "fluids," which I imagined was a nice word for blood. No wonder my breast still hurt like hell. The plan was for that last week to be a targeted radiation just to the cavity to make sure nothing even entertained the idea of setting up residence there. Whatever it took.

I just put my head down and got through it. Having to go to the cancer center every single day kept my schedule so full that it served to help the time pass more quickly.

By the end, the skin over my entire left breast was cracked and raw, and the area under my armpit and all the way through to the back of my shoulder had deep burns. I was practically buzzing. My heart was wonky or my breast was hurting or it was heartburn. It was hard to tell because everything in the general area was f-ed up. I was trying to wean myself off the meds, and every night I thought I was going to need that second half Ativan, but every night by the time the first one kicked in, I didn't care.

My last day fell on a Monday in October. Catherine was out of school, so I brought her with me. It was fun showing her the daily routine I had kept up over the previous few weeks. I said hello to the receptionist and introduced her to Catherine before she waved us back to the changing and waiting room. She stayed in the main room, watching the fish in the aquarium as I took off my top and threw on a gown over my jeans.

When I finished changing, the radiation staff was already ready for me. Saying hello to Catherine, they seemed happy to have a visitor and cheerful about it being the last day. We showed Catherine the mold they had made of my back and shoulders, holding me in the exact same position day after day. It was placed on a metal table under the hulking x-ray machine.

The smaller circular arm of the machine that faced the patients was covered in stickers that the staff or patients had placed over time. I had placed my own early in the process and pointed it out to Catherine. It was a sticker an artist we had met together at the King's Mountain Art Fair early in the fall had given us, and she smiled when she saw the brightly colored pastoral scene with the horse placed on the machine.

"You brought one today, too, remember?" Catherine said.

"Oh, yeah!" I said, fishing it out of my purse. It was small, about the size of a quarter, with a blue butterfly opening its wings above the word Believe. "Why don't you put it on?" I handed it to her and she nodded, looked carefully, and placed it in just the right spot. Then they took her safely into the viewing area while I lay down on the table and was raised and positioned correctly.

While the mechanical arm whirled around and spun into position, it finally rested above me, and I looked right at the sticker Catherine had just placed as if she had known it would fall right in front of my eyes. Believe. I did.

I listened to the instructions called over the speaker system as they had done every day for the previous six weeks telling me to take a deep breath, hold it, then breathe. Suddenly a high voice came over the speakers and said simply, "Hi." The surprise of Catherine's voice on the intercom startled me almost to a laugh, and I had to concentrate to keep still so we didn't have to do it twice. Then after the final position, Catherine's voice gleefully filled the room through the speakers again. "You did it!"

We were congratulated all around, and I was presented with a Three Dots pin, a gift of solidarity from a woman who had been through the process herself symbolizing the tattoos that were left on my body. She had three, I had two, and we both carried the marks with us.

That afternoon we saw the doves again.

At our house in Boston I had heard them in our yard, mostly on the nice days when I would walk out under the trees. In our first Woodside house, the owner kept four beautiful white doves in the aviary with the hens, where I could hear them continually cooing. In San Carlos I always heard them on the daily walk to the park with Maverick, and eventually a pair came to feed regularly on our deck. Here on Manzanita I heard them only occasionally at first, then I saw a flock cross the road at the end of the property in front of me one day. That afternoon I saw a huge flock resting in the trees around our house. They seemed to be trying to navigate around a big group of woodpeckers who had also taken up residence in the soft old trees because they would settle on a few trees then all move together in a long swooping flight and come back to settle again. It was a massive, beautiful, and strong flock, and they flew as a group right over the house several times. There were hundreds of them.

CHAPTER 24

It's a Wrap

November

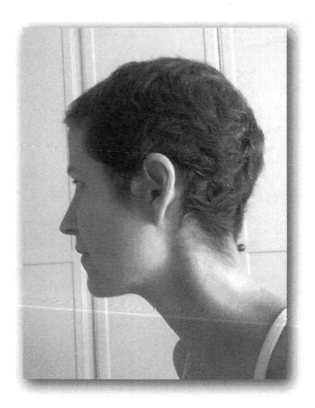

LATER THAT NIGHT, looking into the mirror at my growing hair, almost a legitimate pixie, I exclaimed excitedly to Scott, "Look, I'm about at the stage of that news reporter! I could almost walk around like this, yeah,

I'm a bad ass news reporter covering Iraq, and I cropped my hair because my eyes are beautiful and I just can't be bothered."

He laughed. "It's like a real haircut. I mean, you could probably go to a concert or something and no one would think twice."

And that's how it felt. The last step was finally being able to give up my wig. The hair growing in was gray—not like the handful of silver strands that had dotted my hair before but a flat, ashy gray as if the individual hairs, as thin and wispy as a baby's, lacked any pigment at all. The back and sides had grown slightly longer than the front and started to curl.

I texted Shelley.

Aime: I'm thinking it's almost time for me to ditch the wig.
Shelley: Really? That's a huge step!
Aime: I think so. Want to see a pic?
Shelley: Absolutely!
Aime:

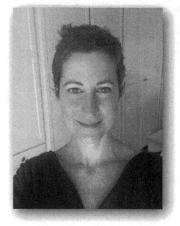

Shelley: OMG

I recoiled. I guess it did look a little weird. A full fifteen minutes passed before she followed up with another text.

Shelley: You look beautiful. You are always beautiful. But it will make a strong statement and you will have to be prepared to handle the reaction from that statement.

What? I thought, incredulous. What was going on? How could she say something like that to me? She had been so supportive all this time, and I couldn't understand how something like hair could illicit this kind of reaction from her. She had tried to walk it back, but her explanation only seemed to clarify what her real feelings were, and those were, it's shocking and it's not your best look.

Then after a day or two I started to realize what was going on. What Shelley had done that was so right during the chemo months was to let me live in a bubble, a slight denial or defiance of reality that allowed me to pretend everything would be all right. For a few hours once a week I was able to act as if none of this was really that bad. But now I knew I didn't need the bubble anymore. I was finally ready to accept things and love myself anyway, maybe even forgive myself for this. I could acknowledge that yes, this was wretched, forgive myself for my body's failure, and be grateful for its redeeming strength.

The price of being vulnerable is that sometimes putting myself out there left me open to other people not being in the same place as me. It was really painful, but it was one of the most important parts about finally growing up and accepting people and myself for who we were. No matter what anyone thought or what anyone else's reactions would be, I was ready. I was ready to face the facts and show the world who I really was and what I had overcome.

I made an appointment with Gretchen, a new stylist, because I needed a color expert, and I was not going back to the poor guy who had butchered the last bit of what I considered my real hair. So I had an initial consultation and we devised a plan. I had a couple of weeks to sit on the idea and get used to it. The cut and color was scheduled for exactly twelve weeks post-chemo.

The bottom line was the people who knew me knew what I was going through. They might not have thought about it every minute, but they knew that my hair was a wig. So if they were shocked by the new super short hair, they'd get used to it.

I was a beautiful woman. I'd been through some terrible shit. I was coming out of it on the other side strong and victorious. Why should I have to keep hiding behind my wig? What my hair would say is that I was a winner. I had won. I was strong.

I did not have to conform to anyone else's notion of perfection because I was perfect the way I was.

Then I was browsing chat rooms about hair regrowth looking for any styling ideas or what other people had done with their "chemo curls," a topic that periodically overtook my thoughts, and I came across a note about wigs. It said that particularly for children with cancer, wigs might suggest that there was something wrong about their new appearance. It said they should be encouraged not to bother with them because not wearing a wig was a way of telling others around them to be gentle. That floored me. All my cheery texts, and my own wig, and hiding out until I was having good days was sending the people around me the message that I was breezing through this. That it was easy somehow. Many people didn't even know or might have forgotten what I was going through.

When I was asked to drive on a field trip or to volunteer for something or was given an eye roll about something I had missed, how could I blame them? I had made a choice to hide my vulnerability, so no one knew. No one. No one knew the depth of my pain. I had made a choice to carry it alone, only sharing bits and pieces with others in a controlled way.

So my hair—that short pixie that looked so "OMG" shocking—was just a fraction of what my body had gone through. It was the least of it. And maybe it was my way of saying, "Yes, I did this and it was hard core. You have no idea."

I felt like I was shedding. I was standing up tall, and things that I no longer needed in my life were falling away. I had shed the cancer, some extra pounds, some extra baggage in my life, and all of my hair. It was like Maverick's winter coat. It took so much work to pull the rake over and over through his fur to get the downy second layer out, but once it was done, he looked and felt so much better, so cool and light and free, and so would I.

The day of my cut and color came, and I sat down in Gretchen's chair and pulled off my wig for the first time in public.

"Okay, let's do this," she said with a smile. We did the color first, and it was such a relief to see the gray strands transform into a nice chestnut with a touch of amber. Gretchen then kept up a steady chatter as she quickly snipped away the soft curls from the back and sides, making a tight clean cut up the back and around my ears. She didn't touch the top at all; she didn't need to as the strands barely touched the top of my forehead.

It all seemed to be going all right until I saw pieces of hair on the floor that were close to an inch long. It reminded me of all the times I gazed longingly into the mirror measuring hairs and trying to decide if they had grown. That inch on the floor represented months of angst.

For many people just the act of losing their hair would be traumatic. Imagine your hair being cut against your will, then remaining bald for months and watching the regrowth come in painfully slowly. The growth is like the hair of a baby or a very old person. I imagined that's why it came back that gray color—and why I felt like I was eighty. That in itself would have been more than a lot of people could handle. But I did, I handled it because there was no choice, and the truth of it was it wasn't even close to being the biggest concern of mine. I hardly ranked it in the top twenty.

I wiped away a few tears as she finished the cut. She gracefully handed me a tissue. "I know. It stinks. But I promise. We'll make it pretty."

And she did. By the time I walked out of there, it actually looked like an intentional haircut. It wouldn't have been my first choice of a style, but it could have been someone's. I shook with nerves and pulled into a Starbucks, craving a sandwich and a green tea lemonade. I hesitated in the car for a minute before I got out.

I texted Lea.

Aime: Can I go out of the house like this?

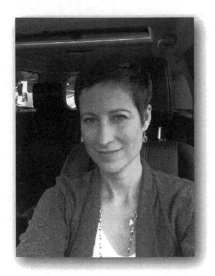

Lea: Of course!! It's adorable. You can totally pull it off. Throw on some cool sunglasses and you'll be mistaken for a movie star.

Aime: I have the wrong sunglasses with me... I think I just need to do this.

Lea: The color is perfect. Looks just like your natural color. Go for it!!

Aime: I like the color. Ok. I'm nervous, but I'm going to act like I'm not. I'm just a short hair girl—it's strong. Ok.

Lea: To me it looks like you want it that style. Channel Anne Hathaway/Halle Berry.

Aime: Yep. I'm in here—it's no big deal. It's not my regular Starbucks anyway ☺

Lea: Good. You'll get used to it and won't even think about it.

I made it back to the car with my green tea in hand and texted her another photo as proof with a huge grin on my face.

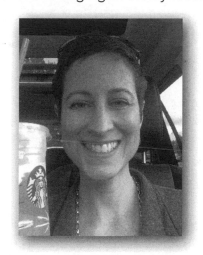

Lea: You look a lot happier now!! Congrats!!

After so many months of wearing a wig and hiding my bare head, it felt as if I were walking around missing a crucial article of clothing, like my pants. But I had made it through a Starbucks run unscathed.

I remembered one of my friends in college saying that he could tell if I had a boyfriend or not by the length of my hair because he had noticed my habit of cutting it short after a breakup. This was like the ultimate breakup from the past, from my old self.

I walked into school for pickup and didn't run into any close friends but got a couple of "Wow, cute cut!" comments from some of the other moms.

"I love that cut," said a mom from another grade that I didn't know. "When did you do it?"

"Today. Just now, actually," I said, running my fingers over the smooth sheared back and bare neck self-consciously.

"Wow, what made you take the plunge?"

"It was time for a change." I smiled, feeling a little lighter.

Only one mom sort of stood and gaped for a moment, but I gave her the benefit of the doubt and hoped she was just trying to place me.

Wesley spotted me, grabbed his friend Bennett, and ran over. He did a little double take at my hair and grinned.

"Is it okay?" I asked quietly, not wanting him to feel embarrassed by the change.

"It's good." He nodded and we all started to walk out.

"I like the new do, Mrs. Card," Bennett said to me. I laughed because it sounded natural coming from Bennett. Somehow it wasn't strange that a nine-year-old boy would notice his friend's mom's hair and also politely comment on it—because it came from him. Nine going on thirty.

In the parking lot Ellen Atwood saw me and hugged me and said, "Oh, it's so cute. I'm so happy for you!" We talked for a minute and Jackie's son James's nanny, Ashley, walked by.

"Aime, I love your hair. It's really cute!" This meant a lot to me coming from her, a beautiful blonde twenty-something who was always put together with the latest trends.

The three of us talked for a while, and I asked Ellen if she was going to the Random Acts of Flowers benefit that night that a fellow school mom of ours was putting on at the Menlo Circus Club. Scott was out of town and I was going solo, sitting with my friend from Woodside, Sarah Park, and a few other ladies whose husbands also couldn't make it.

"Oh, I can't, I have a conflict. Are you?"

"I am. I'm debating whether I can go with this hair or not." I was thinking I might cave and put the wig back on.

"Oh, you can definitely do it! Everyone will be telling you how cute it is. It'll be like a coming out party!"

I picked up Catherine, and when she got in the car she grinned and gave me two thumbs up. By the time we all got home I had a quick turn-around to get dinner on the table for the kids and myself in cocktail attire.

I sent a quick text to Scott along with a picture. "I'm out," I said.

He responded right away. "It's good. It looks like a real cut. Cool."

Jackie called to check in. "How did it go today?"

"It was fine. I'm happy. I think I'm really done with the wig," I said, pondering over my reflection in the mirror while I turned my head side to side.

"I heard from Ashley that it's super cute," she said.

"I'm just debating about tonight. Can I go to the benefit like this?" I thought for dressier events I might keep the wig on hand, but the thought of covering myself up already again seemed wrong somehow.

"Of course! Send me a picture if you're worried. You know I'll tell you the truth. I'm dying to see anyway!"

I got dressed and did my makeup, and following Ashley's advice, popped on a few false lashes even though my own had grown in pretty well by then. Overall, I thought the effect was pretty good and sent a selfie to Jackie.

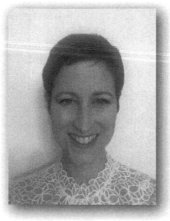

255

"What do you think?"

"Aime. It's beautiful. You look beautiful. I'm so happy for you. Yay!"

She gave me the courage to go out the door, without my wig, to a benefit where most of the women I knew would be attending looking their best.

The Circus Club looked beautiful all lit up at night and sparkling next to the cropped grass of the polo fields. I walked in and gave my name at the desk, looking in toward the party already in full swing. I took an offered champagne glass and spotted Shelley with Sarah and a circle of friends from Woodside and Episcopal. I joined the group, and suddenly a chorus of cheers and compliments showered down on me.

A few moments later Shelley pulled me aside and whispered, "It's beautiful, really. You're beautiful."

"Thanks," I said. And I meant it. I appreciated her for all she had done for me and the particular way that she had helped. Everyone brought something different to the table, and Shelley had brought me exactly what I needed when I needed it. I couldn't expect her to change as soon as I needed to. I could only be grateful for what she had given me then.

Some "friends" bail right at the beginning. Some start strong and then fade away when things get ugly, some heroic friends seem to step up the most in a tragedy, then back away after. Then there are a very rare one or two who remain steady throughout. It doesn't really matter who each person is. I've only every really gotten in trouble with friends when my own expectations are out of whack. People tell me who they are, and it's my job to listen and to love them for that. It's unfair to expect anyone to be otherwise.

We all sat around the table together, enjoying dinner and each other's company, and then the program began. The premise behind the charity was simple—taking flowers from weddings or events that would normally be thrown away, but still had plenty of life left, and re-purposing them in smaller bouquets to give out at hospitals and nursing homes. The staff at the hospitals would guide the group to give the flowers to a person who might need a little boost of happiness. A random act of kindness.

Sitting in a dark room at a table surrounded by friends, I was able to reflect. Tonight for me was not just about the hair. It meant that I was finally becoming free and ready to move forward. And I could gradually start to shift my focus from my own care to the world around me where there was a lot of pain, yes, but also so much love.

When I got home, I saw that Lea had posted one more message on Facebook for me.

Thank you, thank you for all of the thoughts and prayers for Aime. Her treatments are complete and her prognosis is fantastic. She stormed through and never backed down during this battle. Cancer schmancer. She didn't lose a step and continues to be fabulous while now rocking a short hipster do. Love you Aime!!

I did everything they told me to do, and they told me to do it all. Four rounds of AC followed by twelve rounds of Taxol, two surgeries, six weeks of radiation and then starting Tamoxifen for a program that will last years. I think I scared them. My age, stage two, grade three, lymph involvement, two young children at home—they threw the book at me. How many times did I hear the phrase "the combination of the pathology report and your age indicates aggressive treatment"?

I had been through so many emotions, anger being prominent among them. And sometimes that anger helped pull me through. Through the darkest days of feeling like my soul had been sucked out of my body while I sat catatonic on the couch, watching colors and light flash across the television screen in almost indecipherable patterns...like I imagined a cat might do.

But then, little by little my strength had begun to return and I would have a couple of almost normal days before I voluntarily flooded my body with chemicals again. Toxic chemicals, life-saving chemicals. It was the height of contradiction, or irony, that I would have to almost die to give myself the best chance to live.

I was not the same person anymore. I didn't look like it, certainly didn't feel like it, and was not sure I even wanted to be it. One of my biggest fears besides the cancer returning was that I might not change. That I might not learn any lessons. That I might fall back into my old life. I needed to step forward.

Scott got home the next night. I felt like celebrating, so I picked up some steak at Roberts along with a medley of squash, zucchini and root vegetables to make the dinner we all agreed was the family favorite. We bustled around the kitchen, Scott putting the steak on the grill while I chopped and threw the veggies into a stir fry. Catherine and Wesley leaned against the counter, talking with animation about their days.

After dinner we cleared the table then stayed in the kitchen listening to a new playlist Scott had created. Uptown Funk came on, and we all got up and danced together, the kids shrieking with laughter at our "old fashioned" dance moves.

"Let me play my favorite song," Wesley said, grabbing Scott's phone to find it.

Suddenly the room filled with an electronic music that we used to call Techno but he called Dub-Step. Wesley busted out some very professional robotic dance moves that left our jaws hanging in surprise.

"Where did you learn that?" Scott asked him.

He let out a high peel of laughter and turned red in the face before he sputtered, "In the bathroom!"

Catherine joined his raucous laughter and shouted, "So that's what you were doing in there!"

Eventually and in no hurry, we quieted them down and got them to bed, then Scott and I settled into the patio chairs. I looked out over the darkened yard down toward the creek that ran under the horse bridge. The tree guys had taken down three from our view but for some reason had decided to leave my favorite, trimming two of the heaviest branches instead. We had both survived.

Maybe in some strange way I needed cancer. It was gut wrenching to think of it, but I had to embrace the possibility. If someone asked me in a survey in that moment to describe my perfect night, it would be that one. That might not have been my answer the year before. I had cooked a plain and healthy meal without the typical stress or constant chatter in my brain counting all of the ways it could be better. I cleaned up after without being annoyed with the circular task of dishes again. I was glad to be able to do these things because I could. And I knew what it felt like not to be able to. I was strong enough to feed my own family and wash my own dishes. So the ritual of the feeding and caring for my children and husband became joyful, and it transformed an ordinary night into something magical. A gift.

I thought of how I called Scott a simple man, with the basic things he needs to be happy. When it boiled down to it, I realized that I am a simple woman too. I love my family. I like to spend time with real friends that I can trust, I like to leave things a little better than I found them and to feel like I am contributing something positive to the world. Not something big and splashy but something good. Like a kind word at just the right time, or a smile.

In this quiet hour Scott and I looked back on where we had been and where we were going, all the things that now seemed different for us, and how our priorities had shifted. We agreed that it was time for us to go back to the place where we belonged—to our house, to our old friends and family, to the seasons and cadence of life that we understood. All the other stuff—the incremental career boosts and the competition for power, money, and status—didn't matter.

We were lucky. We had a great life. A full life with adventure and joy and tears. A life that it was possible we were just halfway through. In that moment we decided it was time to quit struggling for improvement and to realize that this was enough. We were enough. We had enough. We had done enough. And life—just living, laughing, and being together—was all that we needed. It was beautiful in its simplicity. It was love.

Acknowledgements

My HEART IS filled with gratitude for all of the support I received through-out this journey from the patchwork quilt of people that were con-nected to me somehow. I wrote most of these pages either during my treatment or soon after in the raw stages of healing, many lines even reaching through the fine mist of pharmaceuticals. After a couple of edits, I had to stop and let the words speak for themselves, because while they might not reflect my heart after some distance, they caught my true feelings in that moment, and that, for better or worse, was the point.

In the writing of this book I have the following people to thank, because they each contributed in an essential way.

Scott, for supporting me without question through all the hours spent banging out the stories on the computer, and so often reach-ing for my phone in the night, its bright light filling the dark room and waking you as I tried to capture a thought floating through my mind before sleeping. Thank you for letting my spirit be free and for catch-ing me when I fall.

Catherine and Wesley, for forgiving the late dinners and messy house while I tried to recover and buried myself in the writing of this book. Your love, joy, and courage continues to inspire me to strive to be the best version of myself that I can.

Shena, for encouraging me to turn my disjointed ramblings into something real. I had to follow the wave where it took me, and hope that it might eventually be helpful to someone. Kirsten, for reading every word of the most inflated draft, being a constant sounding board, and cheering me on in so many ways. Holly, for reading it first and providing immeasurable guidance as a friend and mentor. Lea, for having my back, and for always taking care of me. Emma, for believing and telling me I could do this even though you were always the better writer. Dad, Fronda, and Rob, for supporting me in so many ways, even when the burden weighed equally on you.

Kathy, Diane, and Laura, may your words be as helpful to others as they were to me. Thank you for letting me share them.

Special thanks goes to my editor, Meghan Ward – This book was such a mess when I gave it to you, but you patiently took it, helped it, and coached me to make it better. Little comments you made or questions you had about the "characters" caused me to examine things I hadn't understood and worked better than therapy ever could.

And to all my other loved ones finding themselves mentioned in these pages, thank you for the role that you played in my life. Thank you for letting me use the part of the story that we shared, and often even your words as best I remember them. Each of you in your own way contributed to my strength and healing, and I hope in turn, to the strength and healing of others along their own journey.

As of the publication of *And Beneath It All Was Love*, Aime Alley Card is a two-year breast cancer survivor. A mother of two, she lives with her family on the North Shore of Boston, Massachusetts.

The editor of the *LifeSiliconValley* blog, Card is currently working on a historical novel based on true events that took place in her hometown of Nashville, Tennessee.

Made in the USA
Middletown, DE
07 March 2016